Body Contouring Surgery after Weight Loss

Jeffrey L. Sebastian, M.D.

Joseph F. Capella, M.D.

J. Peter Rubin, M.D.

Addicus Books
OMAHA, NEBRASKA

An Addicus Nonfiction Book

ISBN 1-886039-18-6
ISBN 978-1-886039-18-6
Illustrations by Jack Kusler
Typography by Linda Dageforde
Cover design by Lightbourne.com

This book is not intended to serve as a substitute for a physician. Nor is it the authors' intent to give medical advice contrary to that of an attending physician.

Library of Congress Cataloging-in-Publication Data

Body contouring surgery after weight loss / Jeffrey L. Sebastian ...
   [et al.].
       p. cm.
    Includes index.
    SBN 1-886039-18-6 (alk. paper)
    1. Obesity--Surgery. 2. Surgery, Plastic. 3. Liposuction.
I. Sebastian, Jeffrey L., 1967-   .
RD540.B64 2006
617.9'52--dc22   2005031977

Addicus Books, Inc.
P.O. Box 45327
Omaha, Nebraska 68145
www.AddicusBooks.com

Printed in the United States of America
10 9 8 7 6 5 4 3 2 1

Contents

Introduction

If you are among the many people who have changed their lives by losing a significant amount of weight, whether through surgery or diet and exercise, you know firsthand the determination and dedication it took to accomplish this tremendous achievement. You may even have experienced massive weight loss by shedding a hundred pounds or more.

If you have accomplished this, your diabetes and high blood pressure have probably resolved, and you no longer require a handful of medications. However, you may now be wondering what to do about all the excess skin that hangs from your body—skin that causes rashes and makes it impossible to find clothing that fits well. You may be embarrassed to go to the gym or may continue to see yourself as fat in the mirror. If so, this book will serve as an important guide to the powerful options that are available with body contouring surgery.

In the last few years, plastic surgeons have seen a dramatic increase in demand for body contouring procedures following massive weight loss. This demand has led to refinement in technique and remarkable innovation to address some of these very complex problems. Using modern surgical principles, plastic surgeons can now choose from an array of procedures that lead to dramatic improvements. Many of these newer techniques can also be applied to individuals interested in improving the shape of their body, which may be showing the after-effects of pregnancy, aging, or milder degrees of weight loss.

In navigating all the information available on the Internet, television, and through word of mouth, you may find yourself confused and looking for answers to key questions: When will I be ready for surgery? What are my options? What is a body lift? What is recovery like? Will my insurance cover this? What important safety issues should I be aware of? *Body Contouring Surgery after Weight Loss* will provide answers to these important questions, as well as others, and help guide you on your journey to better health and improved quality of life. Achieving the body shape that you deserve and expect following weight loss can now become a reality.

*"The most challenging body contour patients
are those presenting after massive weight loss.
Modern body lifting is an exciting frontier for plastic surgeons.
The results can be dramatic and fulfilling…"*

— Ted Lockwood, M.D. (1945-2005)

Acknowledgments

I am indebted to my patients for their trust and for all they have taught me. In particular, I would like to thank the patients presented in this book who were selfless in openly and honestly sharing their personal experience in order to help others.

I am grateful to have worked with two very talented co-authors, Joseph F. Capella, M.D. and J. Peter Rubin, M.D. Their experience, knowledge and dedication has allowed this book to become a unique and important resource. As a clinical psychologist specializing in bariatric patients, Dr. Leslie Seppinni has also provided valuable input.

I would like to thank the editorial staff at Addicus Books for their expertise, diligence and patience in putting this book together. In particular, I would like to acknowledge Rod Colvin, Graciela Sholander, Susan Adams, and Jack Kusler.

My fellow authors and I thank Dr. Ted Lockwood, a pioneer in body contouring surgery, who set forth sound surgical principles and techniques, allowing for modern-day body lifting surgery to be done safely with predictable and long-lasting results. He has inspired countless plastic surgeons to constantly strive for better aesthetic results.

Lastly, this book is dedicated to my wife Quynh and to my family who have always provided unwavering love and support.

Jeffrey L. Sebastian, M.D.

I would first like to thank my wife Carlyn for her patience and support of my professional and educational endeavors, especially during this very special time with our first child, Lucas. I would also like to thank my father, Dr. Rafael Capella, for his encouragement and many helpful suggestions. My interest in the field of body contouring after massive weight loss is largely the result of my father's commitment of over twenty-five years to the practice and study of bariatric surgery.

I would like to acknowledge my colleagues, Drs. Sebastian and Rubin. It has been a pleasure working with them on this important project. Finally, I would like to thank the entire staff at Addicus Books, in particular, Graciela Sholander and Rod Colvin for making this book a reality.

Joseph F. Capella, M.D.

I would like to thank my wife, Julie, and my daughters, Eliana and Liviya, for their inspiration and steadfast support of my educational activities. I would also like to thank my patients for the privilege of being part of their weight loss journey. It has been a great honor to work with my two co-authors, Dr. Jeffrey Sebastian and Dr. Joseph Capella, who are dedicated to progress in the field of body contouring. Finally, this work could not have been possible without the tireless efforts of Rod Colvin and the staff of Addicus books.

J. Peter Rubin, M.D.

CHAPTER 1

Body Contouring after Weight Loss:
An Overview

Remember the moment you stepped onto the scale and discovered that you'd finally achieved your weight loss goals? Losing a hundred pounds, two-hundred pounds, or perhaps more was no easy task. Congratulations! You made an important decision to improve your health. It took time, courage and a deep commitment. You were, no doubt, exhilarated over your accomplishment. But you may not have anticipated that the weight loss would leave you with excess skin over various regions of your body. You may even feel discouraged when you look in the mirror and realize that you do not look as good as you feel. Excess skin may also be causing considerable difficulty with hygiene and feelings of shame in social situations or even during intimate moments. Although your body may now be much smaller, you are forced to buy oversized clothing to hide the large folds of skin. There may be constant skin irritation, recurrent skin rashes, infections or back pain due to the weight of hanging skin.

No amount of exercise or healthful living will restore elasticity to your skin. However, there is a surgical option for removing the excess skin. It's called body contouring surgery.

WHAT IS BODY CONTOURING SURGERY AFTER WEIGHT LOSS?

Body contouring is plastic surgery designed to correct specific abnormalities or irregularities in the shape of the body. These are procedures that are aimed at restoring contour, proportion, and skin tone.

Although body contour abnormalities following massive weight loss can potentially involve almost every part of the body, it is often unpredictable as to which area will be affected the most and to what degree. There is a wide spectrum of unique post-weight-loss deformities that can be encountered, and, often the magnitude of problems exceeds what surgeons have traditionally addressed with plastic surgery.

For those who have lost more than fifty percent of their excess weight, body contouring surgery will remove significant amounts of excess skin and sagging fat from various regions of the body; these surgical procedures may include tightening underlying tissues and performing liposuction to remove local fat deposits. Often, an individual can qualify for a number of surgical options that cover multiple body areas.

Furthermore, body contouring surgery after massive weight loss can produce results that improve both psychological and physical health. Being rid of pounds of excess skin can mean not only a dramatic improvement in appearance, but an improved body contour may also mean greater self-esteem and confidence. The benefits to physical health include being able to exercise more easily, which may lead to further pounds being lost or at the least easier maintenance of your hard-earned new weight. You may also be relieved of neck and back pain as well as of rashes and infections that may have developed between folds of excess skin.

SKIN ELASTICITY: WHY WE LOSE IT

Thanks to collagen and elastin, which are fibrous connective tissues, the skin has elasticity. When skin with normal elasticity is pressed, pulled, or stretched, it springs back. Skin that has been overstretched for a long period of time, however, loses its elasticity, similar to a rubber band that has lost its stretch. A number of factors affect the structure of skin over the course of a lifetime.

Significant Weight Loss

Gaining a few pounds and losing them over the span of a few months gives skin the opportunity to adjust to these changes and shrink back into position. But, if you have been obese or overweight for many years, your skin has experienced prolonged tension—it's been overstretched across your entire body for a long period of time. Many

of the elastic fibers in the skin have broken down. The more weight you lose, the greater your chances of having loose skin.

Aging and Genetics

Skin elasticity diminishes naturally in all of us as we age. The older we are, the less elastic our skin becomes. Pinch the skin of a healthy eighteen-year-old, and it springs back immediately. Pinch the skin of a healthy fifty-year-old, and it may not spring back as quickly. Your genes play a role, too, in determining how well your skin springs back, or how much excess skin you're left with after you lose weight.

Skin Type

Your skin type also affects your skin elasticity. People with fair skin have a greater tendency to develop loose skin as they age, regardless of body weight or size.

Sun Exposure

Too much time in the sun will damage the skin, both externally and internally. You may be aware that sun can damage the surface of the skin and cause premature wrinkling, sun spots and even skin cancer. Excessive exposure to the sun's intense rays over time can also cause damage to the underlying tissues in the skin, causing the skin to lose elasticity.

Smoking

Not only is smoking bad for your heart and lungs, it's also bad for your skin. If you smoke, or if you're regularly exposed to second-hand smoke, the nicotine you absorb causes blood vessels to constrict, reducing blood flow to your skin. As a result, your skin is deprived of oxygen.

Smoking also causes collagen, a skin protein important for maintaining good skin elasticity, to break down at an accelerated rate. This results in more wrinkles and looser skin. If you quit smoking you will drastically improve the health of your skin, whatever your current weight level may be.

ARE YOU A CANDIDATE FOR BODY CONTOURING?

Whether body contouring is right for you depends on several factors. One of the criteria for determining whether you are a good surgery candidate is your current weight. Your weight is evaluated according to the body mass index.

Your Body Mass Index

Your *body mass index*, or BMI, is the ratio between your weight and your height. As your weight increases, so will your BMI, and this may negatively affect the results of body contouring surgery. Why? Body contouring is primarily effective in removing an individual's loose, hanging skin. However, it is not effective in producing an improved contour if an individual is still significantly obese. These are not procedures for treating obesity. Contouring surgery will not drastically change a severely obese individual's shape because of the excessive fat that underlies the skin. The closer you are to your goal weight, the more ideal your BMI will be, and this will allow contouring surgery to produce the best possible cosmetic result.

Beyond the contouring issues, however, there are greater health risks for patients who have a high body mass index. There is an increased risk with undergoing anesthesia. In addition there may be healing complications; fatty tissues have relatively poor blood supply, increasing the risk for infections. The risk for forming a dangerous blood clot that then travels to the lungs is also increased.

Is there a specific BMI requirement for body contouring surgery? The guidelines are not etched in stone. A plastic surgeon will consider each person's unique circumstance and decide accordingly; however, many surgeons prefer that patients have a BMI of 30 or less to take full advantage of procedures to restore contour. Many surgeons do not recommend extensive body contouring procedures if the BMI is greater than 35. See appendix A to determine your own BMI.

Other Determining Factors

A number of other factors will determine whether you're a good candidate for body contouring surgery.

- Are you are in good health overall?
- Are you committed to a healthful lifestyle that includes proper nutrition and a fitness routine?
- Can you undergo general anesthesia?
- Are you experiencing post-bariatric surgery issues (persistent nausea and vomiting, stomach ulcers, gastrointestinal bleeding, problems with gallstones, weight gain)?
- Are you financially prepared for the costs associated with body contouring surgery?

Advanced age, sixty-five or older, is not necessarily a limiting factor if you are in excellent health with good exercise tolerance. However, if you are this age, your

3

overall medical condition will require greater scrutiny and may limit your options with regard to extensive or lengthy operations. In general, the best candidates for major body contouring work are age fifty-five or younger.

ARE YOUR GOALS AND EXPECTATIONS REALISTIC?

Following massive weight loss, a crucial determining factor of the success of body contouring surgery will be the establishment of realistic goals and expectations. It is important to recognize that surgery will deliver dramatic improvement but not perfection.

Self-Image and Emotional Issues

The way you view yourself is likely to be negatively impacted by the appearance of and the problems associated with your skin excess. This obstacle to building proper self-esteem and self-confidence will be lifted with body contouring surgery. However, the surgery improves the exterior of your body, it will not serve as a cure-all to any negative attitudes or emotions you have prior to surgery. You may continue to have self-image issues.

Anticipating Scars

Depending on the severity of skin excess, the scars may be quite extensive, sometimes extending beyond the usual boundaries for scar placement in plastic surgery. In the end, the trade-off for significant improvement in body contour, alleviation of medical conditions, and lifting of physical limitations is quite acceptable. But, you must give this careful consideration. With strategic planning, scars are typically placed in areas that are hidden by bathing attire or clothing; this may not always be possible, however. If you should need surgical scar revision, it will usually be delayed for eight to twelve months.

The Recovery Period

The recovery period after body contouring surgery can be substantial. You may have had bariatric surgery performed laparoscopically with very small incisions.

Body Mass Index		
Classification of Weight by BMI		**Health Risk**
18.5 - 24.9	Normal	Minimal
25 - 29.9	Overweight	Increased
30 - 34.9	Class I (Moderate) Obesity	High
35 - 39.9	Class II (Severe) Obesity	Very High
Greater than 40	Class III (Morbid) Obesity	Extremely High

SOURCE: United States Department of Health and Human Services, National Institutes of Health

Unless you suffered a setback from surgery, you probably felt close to normal within a week, having experienced minimal discomfort from the actual surgery. However, due to the length of incisions and tightening of underlying tissues, the recovery from body contouring surgery can be more involved, depending on the type and number of procedures performed. For example, if you have a body lift procedure, you are likely to be in the hospital for at least two days, with another four to six weeks at home for recovery. During this time you may have to wear a special garment that could interfere with your usual clothing and may restrict outdoor activities. You will be advised to avoid direct sun exposure to new scars for a minimum of 6 months but preferably until the scars have faded to your own skin color.

When you return to work, you'll need to schedule half days for the first few days if possible, or take a half-hour nap at midday. If you have a desk job, plan on standing up and stretching your legs at least every hour to help with your circulation and the resolution of swelling.

You'll need to wait at least two to three months to buy new clothing, since your waist will continue to decrease in size and your shape will improve as swelling subsides. In fact, you may lose two or more sizes.

Relapse

As with any plastic surgery procedure, results don't last forever. Age, weight fluctuation, gravity, sun exposure and other factors will, over time, lead to some sagging of the skin. However, following massive weight loss, skin elasticity may be so poor that sagging skin recurs with much greater frequency after body contouring surgery. Maintaining good exercise and eating habits will significantly lessen your chances for this to occur, but additional surgery may sometimes be necessary.

Physical Limitations of Surgery

Although body contouring surgery offers options to reshape your body and establish a more youthful look, there are limitations. In particular, if you have suffered from severe obesity most of your life, your underlying skeletal or bony framework has hypertrophied or enlarged significantly to support the weight of your tissues. In particular, the chest or rib cage may protrude or the hip bones may be prominent. With weight loss, the size of your skeleton will not change significantly. Redraping and tightening the skin and underlying soft tissues with body contouring surgery at times may make bony asymmetries more noticeable. For example, in women, it may pose limits to obtaining the ideal breast shape due to prominence of the rib cage.

Will contouring surgery eliminate *cellulite*, the dimpled or "cottage cheese-like" appearance of the skin? Although tightening the skin through body contouring surgery is the best treatment for improving the appearance of cellulite, it will not make it disappear completely. *Striae*, commonly known as stretch marks, will be eliminated only within the areas of skin removed.

WHEN BODY CONTOURING MAY NOT BE FOR YOU

Some medical conditions, such as heart failure, bleeding disorders, and advanced diabetes, may mean that body contouring is not a viable option for you. A history of vascular disease or lymphedema may also limit your options. Or, if you have scars from previous surgeries that have altered blood supply to your skin, your surgeon may advise against having a specific body contouring procedure and may recommend other procedures for you instead. Financial considerations, discussed in chapter 2, may also be a limiting or prohibitive factor.

BODY CONTOURING: HOW SOON AFTER WEIGHT LOSS?

If you have had rapid weight loss as the result of weight loss surgery, you will need to wait at least several months before having body contouring surgery. Typically, your plastic surgeon will want your weight to be stable for at least three months, and preferably four to six months. "Stable" means a fluctuation in weight of no more than a couple of pounds. On average, individuals who have had gastric bypass reach a stable weight and are evaluated for body contouring procedures twelve to eighteen months following their surgery. Weight loss for those with an adjustable gastric band typically occurs at a slower rate, requiring a longer wait before contouring surgery can be performed. See appendix B for a description of bariatric surgery.

WHY WAIT BEFORE CONTOURING SURGERY?

Allow Your Body Time to Recover

Your body needs time to stabilize or reach equilibrium. During the weight loss period, *metabolism* is altered, and your body may not have the necessary resources for wound healing following major surgery. Your immune system is also likely to be depressed, making you more vulnerable to infection.

For individuals who have had rapid weight loss through weight loss surgery, there may be some degree of malabsorption—the inability to absorb proteins, vitamins, and minerals from food. This is especially true for those who've had gastric bypass surgery or a biliopancreatic diversion. Adequate nutrition is essential for wound healing, and the chance for developing poor nutrition or malnutrition is greater during the rapid weight loss period. See appendix C for nutritional information.

You may also become malnourished if you lose too much lean body mass, which can occur if you are losing weight without exercising. Lack of exercise also leads to poor cardiovascular fitness. With approval from your doctor, you will want to engage in an exercise program. Walking is probably the best form of exercise at first. Later, aerobic exercise and the use of light weights can be included. An exercise program will become a vital component to maintaining your weight long-term.

Overcome Weight Loss Plateaus

It is common to hit a plateau prior to reaching your goal weight. With perseverance and proper guidance, however, you can usually overcome this. Remember, your BMI decreases as you get closer to your goal weight, and this provides greater opportunity to obtain the best possible shape, while decreasing the risks associated with surgery.

Acquire New Eating Habits

As you essentially relearn how to eat during the first few months after bariatric surgery, nausea and vomiting may occur frequently. This can lead to abnormalities in *electrolytes*, which are substances in the blood that help to regulate the proper balance of body fluids. An abnormally low level of the electrolyte potassium, for example, could put you at risk for complications while undergoing anesthesia. Regular follow-up and dietary counseling with your bariatric program is key to your success with long-term weight management and prevention of electrolyte abnormalities.

Allow Time for Skin to Adjust

You will also want to give your body ample opportunity to accommodate any excess skin on its own. Given the elastic properties of skin, there will be some degree of recoil, and this may take three to six months to be fully realized. This recoil capacity, however, diminishes significantly with age and increasing severity of skin excess.

UNDERGOING MULTIPLE PROCEDURES

If you have excess skin in various regions of your body, as do most people who've lost a great deal of weight, you may benefit from more than one contouring procedure. For example, you may have excess skin over your abdomen, but a tummy tuck may not be enough. You may also benefit from a buttock lift and a thigh lift. But instead of performing three separate procedures, it may be possible for your plastic surgeon to perform these procedures in one operation in a procedure referred to

as a body lift. Similarly, you may be a candidate to have a breast lift and an arm lift done on the same day.

The advantage to doing several procedures at one time is you have only one exposure to anesthesia and one recovery period. The result following surgery is also more dramatic, perhaps bringing you closer to your overall goal. However, there is a limit as to how many procedures can be safely performed during one surgery, and your procedures may need to be staged.

STAGING PROCEDURES

Staging refers to the order and timing of your body contouring procedures. In most cases, surgical procedures are best staged—spread out over time, often with at least three months or more between procedures. Two to five operations may be required to address all areas of skin excess. A complete series of body contouring procedures may therefore take one, two, or possibly three years to complete. There are several reasons why surgeries need to be staged.

Safety Considerations

It's natural for you to want to complete the entire body contouring process as quickly as possible; however, your safety is of ultimate concern. Most surgeons set a maximum length of time they feel you can safely be under general anesthesia for an elective surgery. This typically ranges from six to eight hours. As time extends beyond this limit, the length of anesthesia and chance for greater blood loss become a concern. For example, a true total body lift combines upper and lower body contouring procedures, all during one surgery. Such an operation may last ten to twelve hours or longer, and even though the result is immediate and dramatic, the recovery and risk for complications are considerable. Although the total body lift is advocated by some surgeons, it is not widespread.

The amount of surgery that can be performed at one time will depend largely on whether your surgeon is operating "solo." Surgeon fatigue becomes a factor for procedures that are complex, precise and labor intensive. Centers performing multiple procedures in one day to address numerous areas of the body often utilize several surgeons as a team.

Doing major procedures in stages is not only a safer method, but it may lead to overall better results because skin is not being pulled in opposite directions at the same time; this "overstretching" could result in loosening of the skin after the operation.

Achieving a Custom Result

Some procedures, such as the body lift, can bring about improvement in multiple areas, possibly eliminating the need for additional surgery. If there is a need for another procedure, it will become more evident once you are completely healed from the previous surgery. This process is not unlike having multiple fittings for custom-tailored clothing.

Recovery

Following extensive surgery, recovery is also an important consideration. As the number of procedures increases, so does the time necessary for recovery. Your body needs greater resources to heal extensive incisions and a long recovery period may

increase your risk for developing a complication.

Combining certain procedures also significantly reduces your ability to move about immediately following surgery, and movement is important for reducing the risk for complications. As an example, since you rely heavily on your arms for mobility after a tummy tuck operation, performing an arm lift simultaneously could pose a problem.

RISKS OF BODY CONTOURING SURGERY

Every type of surgery has some degree of risk associated with it; it's called *inherent risk*. This includes the risk for developing surgical, medical and anesthesia-related complications. Statistically, certain complications will occur despite taking every precaution and properly performing the surgery.

Unsatisfactory Result

With plastic surgery, there is a risk of having an unsatisfactory aesthetic result. You may feel that the primary objective was not met following a body contouring procedure.

Seroma Formation

Serum normally collects between the raw undersurface of the skin and underlying tissues following surgery. A seroma, or pocket of fluid, forms if this accumulation occurs at a faster rate than your body can absorb it and before the tissues have adequate time to heal or seal together. Despite the placement of surgical drains to prevent this, a seroma can develop after drain removal. This can prevent proper healing of the wound, cause discomfort, or may develop into an infection.

Typically, a seroma is treated in the office by aspirating, or withdrawing, fluid with a needle and applying a compression garment. Some cases require either repeat aspiration, placement of another drain, or surgery to properly treat the seroma cavity. This is one of the most common complications following body contouring surgery.

Separation of the Incision

During surgery, tissue is tightened as much as possible, but despite placement of multiple sutures to provide a strong closure, separation of tissue may occur. This separation is called *wound dehiscence*. Certain areas, such as the lower back, are more prone to this. In most cases, the dehiscence is minor. It is usually treated with dressing changes at home, which may prolong the healing period and may also result in a scar that is more noticeable. This is more common when malnutrition is present.

Recurrent Skin Laxity

Especially following massive weight loss, there is a greater risk for significant skin looseness to redevelop due to damage to the skin from years of stretching. This may result in *scar migration* and may require further surgery to correct.

Skin Necrosis

This condition results from an interruption of blood supply to the skin. The affected area turns black in the process of dying, and then sloughs. In most cases, skin necrosis involves a small area. Treatment of skin necrosis may require additional surgery for removal of necrotic tissue and result in

delayed wound healing. Resultant scars may be more noticeable. Individuals who smoke have a much higher chance for this to occur.

Abnormal Scar Formation

Although the placement and extent of scars will be discussed and agreed upon prior to surgery, on occasion scars may develop abnormally, making them more noticeable, unsightly, or even painful. This includes hypertrophic scarring and keloid scar formation. Additional treatment, including injection with steroid, or surgical revision, may be necessary to improve appearance.

Asymmetry

Most body contouring procedures involve working on both sides of the body. Asymmetry may become more noticeable following surgery, since perfect symmetry is rare in most individuals to begin with.

Suture Extrusion

Most body contouring procedures utilize countless sutures for wound closure. Some of these sutures may be permanent and on occasion are expelled by the body. This may cause delayed wound healing or require surgical removal.

Bleeding

Due to the extensive nature of body contouring surgery, postoperative bleeding may require emergency treatment for evacuation of *hematoma*, the collection of blood under the skin. Bleeding can lead to anemia and, in some cases, blood transfusion may be necessary. Bleeding is more likely to be a problem when a bleeding disorder is present, *anemia* exists prior to surgery, or platelet-altering medications like aspirin are taken within a couple of weeks of surgery.

Infection

Although normally the rate of post-surgical infection is low, 1 to 2 percent, this risk becomes higher as your BMI increases. To minimize this risk, you will be given antibiotics at the time of surgery and, in most cases, after surgery until all of the drains are removed. If you are diabetic, especially with poorly controlled blood sugar, your risk for serious infection is also higher. In some cases, mild postoperative infection resolves with a course of antibiotics. In more serious cases, it could mean hospitalization and a trip back to the operating room. Overwhelming or life-threatening infection is uncommon.

LESS COMMON BUT SERIOUS COMPLICATIONS

Deep Venous Thrombosis (DVT)

Deep venous thrombosis (DVT) refers to a blood clot that has formed in the deep veins of the leg or pelvic area. This may result in swelling and pain in the leg, which may become chronic. There are numerous risk factors for DVT, including obesity and a prior history of blood clots. The real danger with a DVT is developing a pulmonary embolism.

Pulmonary Embolism (PE)

Pulmonary embolism (PE) is a potentially life-threatening condition in which a DVT breaks off and travels to the lung, causing obstruction of blood flow. Following bariatric surgery, PE is a leading cause of death. Following weight loss, the risk for

DVT and PE is significantly reduced. Nevertheless, plastic surgeons are especially concerned about this complication and numerous preventative measures are normally taken. This complication may require hospitalization and treatment with blood thinners for a period of months.

Myocardial Infarction (MI)

The medical term for heart attack, a *myocardial infarction* can occur due to the stress of surgery or anesthesia, sometimes even when preoperative tests are satisfactory. This may result in termination of surgery or a prolonged hospital stay.

Pneumonia

Inadequate deep-breathing can lead to poor inflation of the lungs with subsequent fever and may lead to infection called *pneumonia*. Pneumonia requires treatment with antibiotics and can prolong hospitalization.

THE RISK OF COMPLICATIONS

The risk of major life-threatening complications after body contouring surgery is less than 0.25 percent. Although *mortality* following body contouring procedures after massive weight loss is not out of the question, it is exceedingly rare.

Minor complications occur most often with a frequency that can range from 10 percent to as high as 35 percent with more extensive procedures, particularly when BMI exceeds 30. These complications are centered primarily around wound-healing problems. Although they may prolong treatment and healing, in general they do not adversely affect the final result.

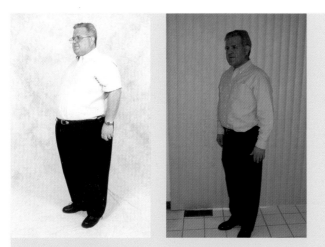

Patient Profile

Name: Edward

Age: 57

Type of WL surgery: Banded Gastric Bypass

Amount of weight lost: 175 pounds

Original Weight: 395 pounds

Current Weight: 220 pounds

How long did it take you to lose the weight after surgery? I lost most of the weight in the first nine months, and lost the balance of the weight in the following three months.

What has changed in your life after losing weight? I am convinced that the weight loss has extended my time here on this earth. Further, my quality of life is so much improved. I can exercise and enjoy taking walks. My outlook has changed. At nearly 400 pounds I was extremely uncomfortable and thought about dying on a regular basis. Now I think about living, and for the first time in a long time I have plans for the future, and the plans include an active lifestyle.

Which body contouring procedures you have had to date? Body lift (abdominoplasty, thigh and buttock lift), chest contouring, arm lift, thigh lift, neck lift.

Over what period of time did you have the body contouring procedures? Approximately one year.

What was most frustrating about the excess skin after the weight loss? Before the body lift the extra skin around my waist was excessive. It would hang over my belt. Slacks didn't fit comfortably; excess skin on my thighs made the legs too tight when I wore the correct waist size. My chest was very flabby. I would not wear a T-shirt of any kind and was never seen without a shirt.

How has your life changed after the body contouring procedures? I am able to enjoy a more active lifestyle. Casual and formal attire fit well and I have a general feeling of well-being. My energy level is much higher. My confidence level has greatly increased.

What is your advice to others, contemplating body contouring? My opening line is, "What are you waiting for?" The weight reduction surgery saved my life, and the body contouring gave me the opportunity to live a new life. Regarding pain, I was fortunate to only experience discomfort; everyone recovers differently. No surgical pain could have ever matched the pain of being morbidly obese.

CHAPTER 2

Choosing a Plastic Surgeon

There are thousands of plastic surgeons in practice across the nation. The question is, which one is right for you? You'll want to make sure that the plastic surgeon who performs your body contouring surgery is well qualified in terms of both training and experience.

Perhaps you already know of an experienced plastic surgeon who has a good reputation. On the other hand, you may not know of any plastic surgeons in your area, and you will need to conduct a more deliberate search.

Word of mouth is often the best way to find a plastic surgeon. If you know others who have had body contouring surgery and are happy with the results, ask them to refer you to their plastic surgeon. You may also be able to get referrals from your bariatric surgeon or your primary care physician.

You can also search for plastic surgeons online at sites such as www.plasticsurgery.org, the official site of the American Society of Plastic Surgeons. Many doctors have Web sites you can browse. After you've narrowed your choices, you may wish to schedule consultations with one or more plastic surgeons. Be advised that most surgeons charge for consultations.

SURGEON QUALIFICATIONS

Any plastic surgeon you consider should be well qualified. Your surgeon needs to have the right training and board certification, as well as experience in performing the procedure you're considering.

Education and Training

Plastic surgery requires years of specialized training, starting with medical school. To become a plastic surgeon, the surgeon must first have graduated from medical school and have a state license to practice medicine. The medical school should be "accredited," which means that the school meets standards set by a national authority for medical education programs.

Once graduated from medical school, a plastic surgeon must complete a minimum of five to six years of additional training in a hospital, where he or she performs surgery. This is often a combination of general and plastic surgery. This period of training is called a residency. Plastic surgery training should be completed in an accredited training program. In some cases this may be followed by a fellowship, which involves training in a specialized area. By the time a surgeon goes into practice, he or she has

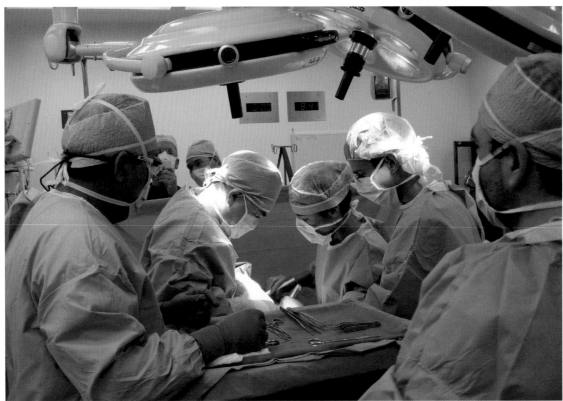

Photo courtesy of Jeffrey Sebastian, MD

A surgical team, led by an attending surgeon, performs abdomen contouring surgery, a procedure which takes two to three hours.

had plenty of real, hands-on experience working side by side with senior surgeons.

Board Certification

Perhaps you have heard that it is important to go to a plastic surgeon who is "board-certified." It sounds important, but just what does it mean? Being board-certified means that after the surgeon has completed residency training, he or she has passed a rigorous written exam, which is followed by an oral exam. These tests are given by a recognized board of senior physicians who oversee the specialty. Once the surgeon has passed these tests, board certification is granted. Any plastic surgeon you consider should be certified by the American Board of Plastic Surgery.

Once certified, a surgeon must update his or her credentials regularly in order to be recertified. This recertification is usually required every ten years. Throughout this period, the surgeon will have received additional training annually through continuing education course work.

Board certification is a completely voluntary process. Surgeons are not required to be certified to perform surgery; however, if you want peace of mind knowing that your plastic surgeon meets important requirements set by an independent board, choose a board-certified surgeon. You can verify a surgeon's certification at the American Board of Medical Specialities Web site at www.abms.org.

Finally, just as with any other doctor, your surgeon needs to be licensed to practice medicine in your state. There's nothing voluntary about licensing—it's required. Your surgeon must have a valid, current license issued by the state's medical licensing board in order to legally practice in the state. Licensing criteria differ slightly from one state to another. If you need further information about a surgeon's licensure, you may check with your state's medical board to learn more about licensing and license verification.

Experience of the Plastic Surgeon

Most plastic surgeons you'll talk to will be well trained and certified. But what about their level of experience with the body contouring procedure you're considering? There are differences between body contouring for cosmetic purposes only and body contouring to address issues after massive weight loss. Most weight loss patients are looking for improvement in function in addition to wanting to enhance their appearance, and this may add to the complexity of the procedures performed. Increasingly, there are plastic surgeons routinely focusing on body contouring in massive weight loss patients. They will often have a working relationship with a bariatric surgeon in the community, which may provide for greater understanding of your specific needs.

How much experience should the surgeon have? We often hear that it's important to ask a surgeon how many procedures he or she has performed. But, it may be difficult for you to know what a "right" answer is. Is it five such procedures a year or is it fifty? To have an appropriate level of experience, most plastic surgeons recommend that the surgeon you choose perform monthly or on a regular basis at least several surgical procedures like the one you're planning.

Finally, a surgeon who is experienced will know how to select the right patients for body contouring surgery. For a variety of reasons, some patients will not be good candidates for the surgery when they first inquire about it, but perhaps they will be later on. An experienced plastic surgeon will know who should and who shouldn't have the surgery.

THE SURGICAL CENTER

Just as it is important that your plastic surgeon be board-certified, it is also

---

Questions to Ask Your Surgeon

- Are you board-certified? By which board(s)?

- Is your surgery center accredited? By which organization(s)?

- Have you ever had your malpractice insurance coverage denied, revoked or suspended?

- Do you have a working relationship with a bariatric surgeon?

- How many body contouring procedures following massive weight loss do you perform monthly?

- Do you have privileges to perform these procedures at a hospital?

- What type of anesthesia will I receive?

important that the surgery center be certified. This is important because a certified surgical center is better staffed and better equipped to perform surgery and to respond to any complications that may arise.

Plastic surgeons perform procedures at a variety of locations. Many work at both an *ambulatory surgery center* (ASC) and at a nearby hospital. Ask where your procedure will be done.

If your surgery will be done in an operating room in your surgeon's office, ask if it is accredited by one of the following organizations: the American Association for Accreditation of Ambulatory Surgery Facilities (AAAASF), the Accreditation Association for Ambulatory Health Care (AAAHC), or the Joint Commission on Accreditation of Healthcare Organizations (JCAHO). You'll find Web sites for these in the "Resources" section in the back of this book.

As with certification, accreditation is voluntary. However, when a facility is accredited by a reputable organization, you can rest assured that it meets the standards set by the accrediting group. This means that the facility, which has been reviewed by the accreditation association, is providing quality and safe care.

CHOOSING THE RIGHT SURGEON

As you discuss possible procedures, ask plenty of questions. Learn as much as you can. Don't be afraid to trust your instincts when you're choosing a plastic surgeon. You need to feel comfortable with the surgeon you choose. You'll also want to feel comfortable with the plastic surgeon's staff. Are they courteous, competent, and sensitive to your needs? Is the office location convenient? If not, are you willing to travel frequently to the surgeon's office? All of these considerations will help you choose the right surgeon for you.

Finally, if you are having general anesthesia, ask if a board-certified anesthesiologist will be present before, during, and after your surgery. You may also want to know what other healthcare professionals will be present during your surgery.

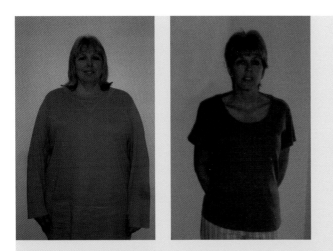

Patient Profile

Name: Wanda

Age: 50

Type of WL surgery: Roux-en-Y Gastric Bypass

Amount of weight lost: 127 pounds

Original Weight: 247 pounds

Current Weight: 120 pounds

How long did it take you to lose the weight after surgery? A little less than a year.

What has changed in your life after losing weight? The big change is in the way I feel. I feel so good. I am free of all the pain I had in my back, legs, and joints when I was overweight.

Which body contouring procedures have you had to date? I have had a lateral thigh lift, buttock lift, and breast lift with augmentation.

What was most frustrating about the excess skin after the weight loss? The most frustrating thing was having rashes and sores form in the folds of skin. The way my clothes fit was also very frustrating. All the excess skin was just generally uncomfortable. It was hard to sit for very long.

How has your life changed after the body contouring procedures? I feel better about myself I and look better. I am more active and outgoing than I ever used to be. I always tell people about my weight loss and my body contouring surgery and that I would do it all over again. I am very happy with the way I feel and about my appearance.

What is your advice to others, contemplating body contouring? My advice is don't wait any longer. You will feel much better after you do it. Find a good, qualified surgeon with a good staff (you will be talking to them a lot). Don't be afraid to ask questions. Go to a support group. They are fun and will help you learn what to do and what not to do.

CHAPTER
3

Your Consultation

By the time you have an initial consultation, you may have already decided on a plastic surgeon. Or, your consultation may be part of your decision-making process. Whichever the case, your consultation is the opportunity to learn from the plastic surgeon as much as you can about body contouring procedures, understanding there may be variations from surgeon to surgeon regarding technique, preference for scar placement and staging of procedures. You also should be able to learn which contouring procedures might work best for you.

Consultations, whether you have two or three prior to your surgery, are opportunities for you to measure the vital "human factor." Having a good rapport with your surgeon will help things go smoothly and make the entire experience much more pleasant.

CONVEYING YOUR GOALS FOR SURGERY

As you and your doctor discuss possibilities, make sure you clearly convey the results you'd like to achieve. Your plastic surgeon will help you understand which goals are attainable. If you're not a good candidate for a specific procedure, you'll be informed; perhaps you'll be given other options.

YOUR MEDICAL HISTORY

Your plastic surgeon will need to know your complete medical history, including any medical conditions, such as diabetes, heart disease, asthma, high blood pressure, anemia, or bleeding disorders. A number of conditions can increase the risks associated with surgery and, thus, limit your body contouring options. Depending on the medical condition, the plastic surgeon may advise against certain procedures.

Your surgeon will also ask what medications you're taking. Some drugs can interfere with surgery and raise the likelihood of complications. This includes recreational (illegal) drug use, which can increase your risk for anesthesia complications. Your doctor may ask you to temporarily stop taking certain drugs, both prescription and over-the-counter, to keep you safe during surgery. Also tell your surgeon if you've ever experienced an allergic reaction to any medications or anesthesia. It is vital that your surgeon know about these before you schedule a procedure.

It is also important to let your surgeon know of any vitamin or mineral supplements you are taking as a result of your weight loss surgery. Your surgeon is also likely to inquire about your current dietary habits and exercise tolerance to gain some insight into your ability to undergo surgery.

If you smoke, let your doctor know. Smoking slows down the healing process considerably and increases the risk of serious complications during and after surgery. At the very least, your surgeon will insist that you stop smoking four to six weeks prior to and after your procedure. Some surgeons may not even consider you a candidate for major body contouring procedures if you smoke, given the significant risk it poses.

YOUR SURGICAL HISTORY

If you've had any surgeries, tell your doctor. In some instances, it may not be possible to perform a procedure because your scars may pose too high a risk of surgical complications.

These are important questions the surgeon will ask:

- Have you had weight loss surgery?
- If so, what kind—gastric bypass, Lap-Band, other?
- How long ago did you have weight loss surgery?
- Is your current weight stable?

YOUR MENTAL HEALTH HISTORY

You should also discuss any significant emotional issues that require treatment or therapy. Depression and anxiety are common but do not prevent you from having surgery. However, your plastic surgeon may request evaluation by a psychiatrist or psychologist, since the stress of surgery may worsen these conditions if they are not properly controlled.

YOUR PHYSICAL EXAMINATION

As part of the consultation, the surgeon will examine you physically. He or she will be examining for the amount and location of skin excess as well as the quality of your skin. The presence of any associated conditions such as skin irritation or rash will be documented. The surgeon will also be looking for any signs of malnutrition, hernia formation, poor circulation or tissue edema, which could affect your healing ability. Existing scars, including those from weight loss surgery or other contouring procedures, will be examined. You may also be weighed.

During your physical exam, the surgeon may have you stand in front of a mirror as he or she discusses how your body will likely respond to contouring surgery. The surgeon may pull up the skin in the regions to be modified by surgery to give you a clearer picture of what results to expect. You'll also be shown where incisions will be made and where scars will be after surgery. You can ask your surgeon to draw the scars with a body marker so you can clearly clearly see their placement.

With your permission, the surgeon will take photographs during the consultation; these photos help with planning and execution of surgery and may be used to obtain insurance coverage by substantiating any medical problems that you may have. To track your progress, these "before"

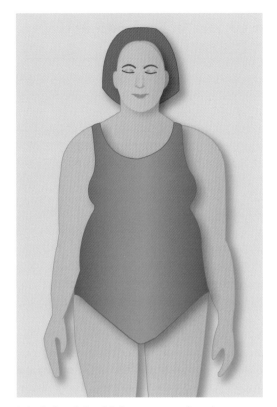

Individuals with "apple" shapes carry weight in their abdomens.

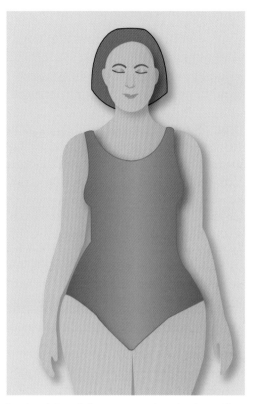

People with "pear" shapes carry weight in their hips and thighs.

pictures will be compared to your "after" pictures, typically taken at least three months following surgery.

BODY SHAPE: APPLE OR PEAR?

People differ according to fat distribution or where the body stores fat. In general, most people fall into one of two categories; *android* or "apple-shaped" individuals have abdominal obesity and more fat in the love-handle area, whereas *gynecoid* or "pear-shaped" individuals carry most of their weight on their hips and thighs. Although men tend to be apple-shaped and women pear-shaped, there is considerable overlap. The shape is important, since it will also determine where problems develop as weight is lost; quite simply, the skin overlying areas that carried most of the fat has been stretched the most and is likely to show the greatest excess.

HERNIA REPAIR

During your consultation, you and the surgeon may discuss hernia repair. Many weight loss patients have hernias, a protrusion of an organ or tissue through a connective tissue defect, usually in the wall of the cavity in which it is normally enclosed.

21

Questions to Ask Your Surgeon

- Are my goals realistic?

- What are my body contouring options?

- Where will I have scars?

- How long will surgery take?

- How would you describe the recovery period?

- What are the risks?

- Do you accept insurance payments?

- Are you a contracted provider for my insurance company?

- Will your office assist with obtaining insurance authorization?

- What is the total cost? Out-of-pocket expenses?

- What are non-insurance payment options?

This is usually evident as a bulge in the area of the belly button or at the site of a previous incision. A hernia may cause pressure, pain or discomfort. It can also pose a danger by leading to strangulation and rupture of the intestine.

Hernias may be present at birth; they can also develop as a result of weight loss surgery. If you have a hernia, your plastic surgeon may be able to repair the hernia during a body contouring procedure, such as a tummy tuck or a body lift. In some cases, this will be done together with a general surgeon or your bariatric surgeon. A strong yet soft screen-like material called mesh may be used for repair. If you have a hernia, ask your doctor during your consultation about this procedure.

ASK TO SEE "BEFORE AND AFTER" PHOTOGRAPHS

During your consultation, your surgeon should be willing to show you "before and after" photos of other patients who have had the procedures you're considering. This is standard practice. Most surgeons will have a collection of photos of other patients who have given permission to have their photos shown to other patients. Although in many cases lengthy scars are unavoidable, you will want to pay attention to overall improvement, symmetry, and scar locations.

Many surgeons are also willing to put you in contact with previous patients who have undergone body contouring procedures. Most bariatric surgery programs have regular support group meetings, where many patients will share their experience with body contouring. Internet chat rooms are also popular forums to share information. These all give you excellent opportunities to hear first-hand accounts of what the surgery was like.

TAKE-HOME INFORMATION

Following your consultation, your surgeon probably will give you written information or perhaps a tape or disk that further describes the procedure for which you are a candidate. These materials usually include instructions to follow before and after surgery as well as office policies on payment. It is important that you review this information carefully; you should not hesitate to call the surgeon's office with any questions.

INFORMED CONSENT

Your decision to proceed with surgery should be a well-informed one. Unfortunately, the practice of medicine and surgery is not an exact science. There are any number of variables that factor into your body's ability to heal satisfactorily. As mentioned, every operation has inherent risk related to surgery and anesthesia. The process of obtaining informed consent involves educating you regarding not only the benefits, but also the risks of surgery. The risks and benefits of your particular operation will be provided, usually in both a written format and through discussion with your surgeon. If you choose to go forward with surgery, you'll be asked to sign an informed consent form. This process of evaluating the risk-to-benefit ratio will be an important aspect of your decision to proceed with surgery.

A WORD ABOUT PRIVACY

Your plastic surgeon has a strong commitment to maintaining privacy and professionalism during the course of your evaluation and treatment. He or she realizes that during the course of your relationship you may be placed in uncomfortable situations, such as having your photos taken to document your condition. Your surgeon and the staff recognize this vulnerability and will treat you with the sensitivity, dignity, and respect you deserve.

As a necessary component of your care, information may be disclosed to other healthcare professionals or your insurance company. However, healthcare providers are legally required to abide by security mechanisms to ensure confidentiality of information that pertains to you, according to state and federal laws, including the Health Insurance Portability and Accountability Act (HIPAA). These privacy rights will be made known to you at your initial consultation.

FINANCIAL CONSIDERATIONS

What are the costs for body contouring surgery? It's difficult to list uniform fees since they will vary across the nation. However, the cost for a procedure is usually the combination of three fees— those for the surgeon, the anesthesia, and the facility. The facility fee will include charges for the operating room, recovery room, and any overnight stay or hospitalization. Additional charges may arise from blood work, other studies, extra days in the hospital, and post-operative garments.

You may be required to place a deposit at the time a surgery date is chosen. Be sure you understand the cancellation policy. Most doctors will ask that you pay the balance of your surgical fees just before your procedure, and you will have to pay a deposit or the balance to the surgery center or hospital prior to admission.

If you have no health insurance, some plastic surgeons will ask that you obtain coverage in case you should require hospitalization in the event of complications. As you know, with any surgery there is always some level of risk involved. Most surgical complications are minor; however, more significant complications, such as infection, occasionally develop.

Lastly, policies regarding payment for *revisional surgery*, or a touch-up procedure, will vary. These procedures are not uncommon after body contouring procedures done following massive weight loss, and

23

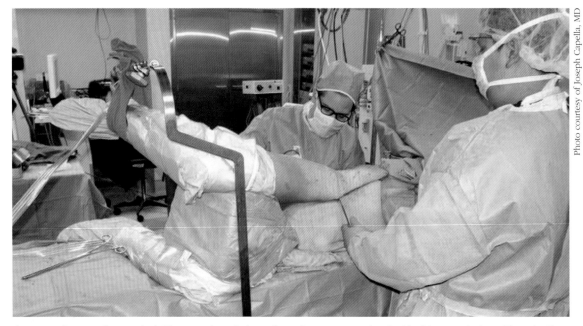

Photo courtesy of Joseph Capella, MD

The surgeon here is perfoming a body lift, a procedure which usually involves a tummy tuck and a lift of the outer thighs and buttocks. The operation takes approximately four hours.

most of these follow-up procedures are unavoidable. You should be familiar with your surgeon's payment policy.

Will Insurance Pay?

You may be wondering if insurance will cover the cost of contouring procedures or if there are other payment options? In determining your eligibility for coverage, third-party payors or insurance companies will make a distinction between body contouring procedures done for cosmetic reasons and those performed for health or reconstructive reasons and thus medically necessary.

Cosmetic Surgery or Reconstructive?

What is the difference between cosmetic surgery and reconstructive surgery? As defined by the American Medical Association (AMA), cosmetic surgery is performed to reshape normal structures of the body in order to improve the patient's appearance and self-esteem. Reconstructive surgery is performed on abnormal structures of the body, caused by congenital defects, developmental abnormalities, trauma, infection, tumors, or disease. It is generally performed to improve function but may also be done to approximate a normal appearance.

Purely cosmetic surgery procedures are not covered by insurance. However, there are times when insurance will cover the cost of body contouring surgery if the procedure is done primarily to treat a health problem or for functional reasons. For example, if you are dealing with rashes, skin breakdown, or infections that develop under folds of excess skin, your insurance provider may authorize treatment since these conditions pose a health risk. You may have difficulty walking due to the size and weight of a large *pannus*, an apron of skin hanging around your waist. Or, if you're having a hernia repair at the same time as a body contouring procedure, insurance may provide some coverage of the fees.

Document Medical Problems

If you are able to document medical problems, you may increase your chances for an insurance company paying for your surgery. For example, you may be able to support your request for surgery coverage if you can provide medical documentation showing that continued use of an antifungal cream failed to treat infection between skin folds. Accordingly, it is important to alert your primary care physician or bariatric surgeon to any problems that you develop as weight loss progresses so the problem can be recorded in your medical records.

Common medical problems that qualify for insurance payments include:

- Chronic inflammation of a large apron of excess skin that hangs below the waist, resulting in pain and hard nodules beneath the skin

- Chronic rash, irritation, infection, chafing on skin surfaces

- Back pain from weight of large pannus

- Difficulty walking

- Umbilical hernia or ventral (abdominal wall) hernia

- Enlarged breasts, associated with back, shoulder, neck pain, headache, bra-strap grooving with pain or ulceration

In general, however, insurance companies are becoming more strict with their requirements. Conditions for coverage will differ between insurance companies; consequently, it is important to check with your insurer for specific requirements. In most cases, the surgeon's administrative staff will help seek insurance authorization.

Other Payment Options

Since insurance coverage for body contouring procedures is not guaranteed, what do you do if insurance will cover only a portion of the cost of your surgery? Additionally, there are a fair number of surgeons who do not accept insurance. This gives them greater freedom to perform the most appropriate procedure without limitations on what is not covered. If you are planning on having extensive reconstruction of your body contour, financial planning is important since cost may be significant for surgical procedures that can be lengthy and require extensive follow-up care.

For procedures that need to be done in the hospital, your surgeon may have negotiated lower out-of-pocket rates with the hospital. Furthermore, many surgeons will offer a discount when more than one procedure is done at one time. In some cases, staging several procedures over time can significantly lessen the cost burden and allow for better financial planning.

There are a number of financial strategies to consider. Financing may be available through your plastic surgeon's office or through a lending institution working with the office. The office administrative staff will discuss financial options with you.

Under the right circumstances, obesity-related medical expenses, such as those for body contouring surgery, may qualify for a tax deduction. Similar to insurance company requirements, qualifying deductions would involve procedures that are medically necessary and not cosmetic. Supporting medical documentation should be obtained. Consult with a certified public accountant or tax attorney for further recommendations.

Finally, financial considerations may weigh heavily on your mind as you consider body contouring surgery after weight loss. Although insurance may provide some coverage, out-of-pocket expenses can be substantial. However, proper anticipation, knowledge, and planning can help alleviate anxiety and make your pursuit of a better body a reality.

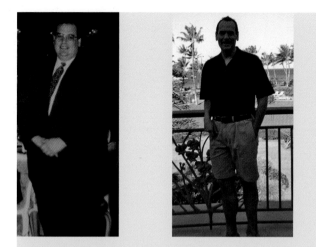

Patient Profile

Name: Peter
Age: 46
Amount of weight lost: 216 pounds
Original Weight: 400 pounds
Current Weight: 184 pounds

How did you lose weight? I lost my weight through diet and exercise.

How long did it take you to lose the weight? I lost most of the weight in about two years time.

What has changed in your life after losing weight? I have more confidence in all aspects of life. I feel much better, with no aches and pains in my joints. Also, I am able to get around a lot easier, have a lot more energy, and can exercise much more. I run three times a week and do weight training three times a week. I never did either before weight loss. I travel weekly for my job and travel is much easier.

Which body contouring procedures have you had? Panniculectomy (removal of skin on the abdomen and sides), chest contouring, inner arm lift, and an inner thigh lift.

What was most frustrating about the excess skin after the weight loss? My weight loss felt incomplete since I still had a lot of flab after getting to a normal weight. This was frustrating since I never felt that I had achieved my goal of looking normal. The flab could be partially hidden in clothing, but I still looked lumpy. I was still very self-conscious. The result was that this was counter-motivating in keeping the weight off. I had the tendency to continually re-gain and re-lose 20 to 30 pounds.

How has your life changed after the body contouring procedures? I now feel complete in reaching my goals of looking normal. It has been very motivating for keeping the weight off, and I have been much more successful than before in not regaining the weight.

What is your advice to others, contemplating body contouring? Find a surgeon who has the experience along with a great understanding of the emotional side of things. Realize that the recovery period may be a difficult time. It was for me. I had a lot of postoperative pain, much worse than I thought it would be, although my surgeon advised me about the pain. Make sure you have the strong support of family or friends to get through what may be an emotionally trying time.

CHAPTER 4

Preparing for Body Contouring Surgery

As with any surgery, body contouring procedures require careful preparation and planning—on the part of your surgeon and on your part, as well. Because your safety will be of primary concern to your plastic surgeon, he or she will consider a number of factors in determining whether you are ready for surgery. Your surgeon will want to have a clear understanding of your overall health—mental and physical—especially if you have had weight loss surgery.

MEDICAL EVALUATION AND CLEARANCE FOR SURGERY

Your health will likely have improved dramatically with weight loss. In fact, serious medical conditions related to obesity are likely to have resolved. Your risk for undergoing anesthesia is also reduced. However, you may still have medical conditions that require ongoing treatment and could limit your options for body contouring surgery.

Your plastic surgeon will likely call on your primary medical doctor (PMD) to help prepare you for surgery. A referral will be made if you do not have a current doctor. You will be asked to obtain a preoperative medical evaluation and clearance for surgery, usually performed by your PMD. This evaluation shows that you are considered an acceptable risk for surgery. It may also contain additional recommendations to further minimize your risk while undergoing surgery.

If your medical problems are complex, you may require further evaluation by a specialty doctor, such as a cardiologist or a pulmonologist.

Lab Tests and Studies

Several routine diagnostic tests may be ordered by your plastic surgeon. The surgeon may refer you to your primary care physician who will order the tests and send results to the plastic surgeon.

Complete Blood Count

The *complete blood count* test, often called a CBC, is the most common test ordered to check for any abnormalities in the blood. A CBC includes a total of thirteen tests; the main portions of the test measures the health of three major blood cells: white blood cell count (WBC), hemoglobin (HGB), and blood platelets. White cells fight infection in the body; hemoglobin carries oxygen to organs and tissues; platelets are essential for clotting.

If you're contemplating body contouring surgery, your surgeon will want to rule out anemia by checking your hemoglobin level. Low hemoglobin means a deficiency of red blood cells resulting in insufficient oxygen delivery to tissues and organs. People with anemia are said to have "tired blood." Symptoms can include feeling tired, weak, and having shortness of breath. For those who have previously had weight loss surgery, there is an increased risk of anemia due to decreased absorption of certain nutrients, such as iron and vitamins. Menstruating women in particular are at risk. Undergoing any major surgery while anemic will increase the chance of your requiring a blood transfusion.

Comprehensive Metabolic Panel

Another blood test, a *comprehensive metabolic panel* (CMP), is actually a group of fourteen separate tests used by physicians to screen and evaluate organ function. Your physician will use this panel to make sure there are no electrolyte deficiencies. Electrolytes are minerals such as sodium, potassium, magnesium, and calcium, which are essential for the body and heart to work properly. For example, a low potassium level could put you at risk for anesthetic-related complications such as irregular heart rhythms. Similar problems could result from a calcium deficiency. The metabolic panel will also measure the level of total protein and albumin in your blood, which are indicators of your nutritional status.

Coagulation Studies

These studies measure your blood's ability to coagulate or stop bleeding. In some cases, you may also have a bleeding time checked, which specifically measures the clotting ability of blood platelets. Abnormalities in these studies may indicate a risk for excessive or prolonged bleeding with surgery. Causes for these problems may include nutritional deficiencies, liver dysfunction, certain medications, and inherited bleeding disorders such as hemophilia.

Vitamin and Mineral Levels

If you have had bariatric surgery, certain vitamin and mineral levels may need to be checked. Specifically, vitamin B12, folate, calcium, and iron may be low after a gastric bypass. With the biliopancreatic diversion, vitamin A can be deficient. Low zinc and vitamin C levels will prevent proper wound healing.

Twelve Lead Electrocardiogram (ECG or EKG)

This test measures heart electrical activity. In evaluating the results, the physician is looking for signs of irregular heart rhythms. It may also indicate signs of past heart attacks. This is a non-invasive test which requires the attachment of twelve electrodes to your chest. An EKG machine measures the electrical currents created when your heart beats and prints out a report for your physician.

Chest X-ray

Typically, your plastic surgeon will want to examine the results of a chest X-ray for potential problems with the heart and lungs. For weight loss patients who have a history of sleep apnea, the surgeon will be looking for evidence of damage to heart tissue. If an X-ray suggests signs of heart enlargement, the surgeon will likely want to investigate further.

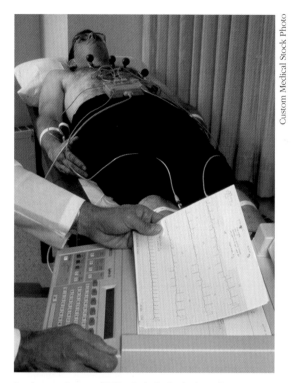

Custom Medical Stock Photo

An electrocardiogram (EKG), which checks the heart for any irregularities, is one of the lab tests required before body contouring surgery.

Mammogram

Women forty years of age or older will need a mammogram that tested negative for cancer within the year prior to the date of planned breast surgery.

Additional Studies

Depending on the results of these standard tests, you may need to undergo further evaluation. For example, an abnormality on an ECG may prompt further investigation with a stress test to determine whether your heart is able to withstand the stress of surgery and anesthesia. Also, based on your medical history, your doctor may require additional testing. Women of child-bearing age may be asked to take a pregnancy test just prior to surgery, to avoid exposing an unborn child to the harmful effects of surgery and anesthesia.

NUTRITIONAL ASSESSMENT

After any surgery, your body needs to be able to process nutrients efficiently in order to heal. Bariatric surgery dramatically affects the way your body processes food and its nutrients. With procedures such as the gastric bypass you are required to take lifelong nutritional supplements, but significant deficiencies of certain vitamins, minerals, or protein may still develop.

Deficiencies may lead to conditions such as anemia, a bleeding disorder, accelerated osteoporosis, night blindness, or neurological disorders. Since some deficiencies will increase your risk for having surgery because they impair your body's ability to heal properly, any such deficiencies must be corrected prior to surgery. If you are planning to have a series of procedures over time, your nutritional state will need to be optimal to allow for proper recovery between surgeries. Regular follow-up with a nutritionist in your bariatric program will allow for monitoring and correction of any deficiencies.

MEDICATIONS YOU'LL NEED

A week or so prior to your surgery, most surgeons will prescribe the medications you will need once you have returned home from surgery. It's a good idea to have these prescriptions filled and waiting for you at home.

31

Pain Medication

A few individuals will be able to get by with just over-the-counter pain medicine, but they will be the exception rather than the rule. Expect to take prescription pain medication for three to seven days—in some instances longer—following your procedure.

Antibiotics

Your doctor may also prescribe *oral* antibiotics as a precaution against infection. If drainage tubes are placed during surgery, many surgeons will recommend taking antibiotics to guard against infection until all of these tubes have been removed.

Bowel Prep

If a hernia repair is part of your planned operation, you may be asked to take a bowel prep in advance of surgery. This typically consists of taking a liquid laxative, which will flush your bowel clear prior to surgery. In combination with oral antibiotics, this will decrease the bacterial count in the colon and reduce the risk of infection. You may also be asked to remain on a clear liquid diet the day before surgery.

Sleeping Aids

In some instances, your surgeon may prescribe a sleeping pill for you to take the first few nights after your procedure. These are safe to take along with pain medication if taken in the prescribed dosages.

Anti-Nausea Medications

On occasion, you may be given anti-nausea medication to be taken as needed as you recover at home.

Stool Softeners

Since narcotic medications may cause constipation, you may be given a prescription for a stool softener for the first few weeks following your surgery.

Vitamins and Minerals

If you have had gastric bypass surgery, you will already be taking a daily chewable multivitamin. Otherwise, your surgeon may request that you begin taking one to ensure that your body has the necessary nutrients to heal. You may also be asked to take extra vitamin C. Anemia associated with bariatric surgery is often treated with iron supplements and injections of vitamin B-12, or in some cases, a medication to boost red blood cell production in your bone marrow.

Since vitamin E may cause excessive bleeding, do not take doses in excess of 400 IU (international units) of it daily for two weeks prior to surgery. You will need to check the vitamin E content of your multivitamin.

MEDICATIONS AND SUPPLEMENTS TO AVOID

It is very important that your plastic surgeon is aware of all medications and any vitamins, minerals, contraceptives, herbs, tonics, or other natural supplements you're currently taking. Some substances found in supplements can cause complications with surgery. This could mean a dangerous reaction to anesthesia or an increased risk of bleeding. Your surgeon will likely instruct you to stop taking any medications containing aspirin or ibuprofen. These drugs can promote excessive bleeding during and after surgery. For pain relief you can take medications containing

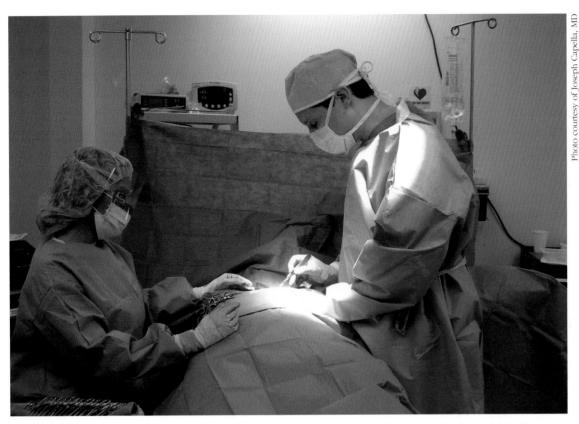

Photo courtesy of Joseph Capella, MD

In the surgery underway above, the surgeon performs an upper body lift, which combines lifts of the arm, upper back, sides, and breasts. The operation takes approximately five hours.

acetaminophen, such as Tylenol. See appendix D for a list of medications and natural supplements to be avoided.

AUTOLOGOUS BLOOD DONATION

If you are not anemic, you are a candidate for *autologous blood donation*. This means that you donate your own blood for potential use during your surgery, eliminating the risk of incompatibility and reducing the risk of a reaction or transmission of infectious agents. Blood is donated within one month of the surgery. The possible need for a blood transfusion will depend on the procedure(s) performed. This is typically a greater consideration for more extensive contouring procedures, such as a body lift.

STOP SMOKING

If you smoke, you'll need to stop smoking completely four to six weeks before your surgery. You must stay away from all forms of nicotine, including cigarettes, pipes, cigars, patches, gums, and chewing tobacco. This includes any significant second-hand smoke exposure. Smoking interferes with healing. Among its many adverse effects, it causes small blood vessels to shrink; as a result, less oxygen—which is vital to healing—is being delivered to the incision site. Smoking also increases your risk of lung problems from general anesthesia.

DIET AND EXERCISE

In preparation for surgery, you will want to be in the best possible physical condition. This will require a commitment to eating a healthful and balanced diet. In particular, protein intake needs to be adequate, typically no less than sixty grams per day. This is often best achieved by keeping a daily food log and developing an awareness of the protein content for various food items.

You should stay well hydrated, preferably with water or non-caffeinated sugar-free, beverages. Minimize your salt intake; a diet high in salt can worsen postoperative swelling. Exercise appropriate for your ability is important to tone your muscles and preserve lean body mass, as well as to boost your cardiovascular fitness. Your body will recover from surgery faster when you are physically fit.

As you think ahead to your recovery at home, prepare or purchase meals, which can be frozen, to last for the first couple of weeks following surgery.

Avoid Alcohol

Do not consume alcohol during the week (in some cases longer) before your procedure. Alcohol thins the blood and can cause excessive bleeding during surgery. It could also pose a danger in combination with anesthetic agents and other medications you will be given.

ARRANGE FOR A CAREGIVER

Before your procedure, you'll need to arrange for a trusted adult friend or family member to take you home after surgery. Since you will have been given heavy doses of pain medication, it will not be safe for you to drive. Your doctor will not release you to a taxi or shuttle service.

Also, be sure you make arrangements for someone to take care of you at home for your first full day and, in some cases, for two or three days. An adult should stay with you at least the first night. If you need assistance with this, ask your surgeon's office to help make arrangements for a home aide or a licensed nurse. If you take care of young children or an elderly relative, you'll need to make other care arrangements.

TRAVEL AND ACCOMMODATIONS

If you must travel a distance to the surgery facility, you may want to avoid the stress of driving very early in the morning on the day of your surgery by staying near the facility the night before your operation. Similarly, staying at a nearby hotel following discharge until your first postoperative visit is an option to consider. Your surgeon's office can provide you with a list of local accommodations.

TIME OFF WORK

You will need time off work after surgery. The length of time you'll need to be off depends on the procedure you're having, how quickly you're recovering, and the nature of your job. With certain procedures, you'll be allowed to return to work as soon as ten to fourteen days after surgery. With others, you'll need a six-week absence.

If your work involves heavy lifting or rigorous physical activity, you may have to wait more than six weeks before you can return. Be sure to talk with your manager or supervisor about your absence well before your scheduled procedure.

TAKING ROUTINE MEDICATIONS

It is important for you to receive preoperative instructions from your surgeon that are specific for each of your medications. If you take prescription medications for medical conditions, your doctor may ask you to keep taking your medicine up to the day before or the day of your surgery. High blood pressure medicine is a good example; most surgeons will ask you to take your medication with a sip of water early the day of your surgery to keep your blood pressure under control. Note, however, that this advice does not pertain to all medications.

It is also important to provide your surgeon with a list of all medications you are taking and their dosage. After your surgery, this information will enable your surgeon to write orders for medications to be taken while you are in the hospital. He or she will also give you specific instructions about resuming your regular medication schedule at home.

FASTING PRIOR TO SURGERY

No matter what kind of body contouring surgery you are having, you will be told not to eat or drink anything after midnight the night before the scheduled operation. Because your stomach takes six to eight hours to empty itself of food, a midnight cutoff means your stomach should be cleared out by the time you undergo surgery. You may consider eating a lighter dinner the night before your surgery and stop eating earlier than midnight.

Having an empty stomach is especially important if you are having general anesthesia because you lose control of several reflex functions. This includes the *gag reflex* that keeps food and stomach acid from rising up in your throat and spilling into your lungs. Serious problems, including a life-threatening illness called *aspiration pneumonia*, can be caused by the aspiration of food particles into the lungs. This hazard can be avoided simply by following your surgeon's instructions to fast after a certain hour.

HYGIENE AND HAIR CARE

You should shower or bathe the evening or morning before surgery with a mild soap or the cleansing agent provided by your surgeon. Avoid body lotions, creams, oils, perfumes, and makeup the day of surgery. Remove any fingernail and toenail polish.

Do not shave or wax hair in areas where you will be having surgery since this will increase the risk of infection. If necessary, shaving of these areas will be done by the medical staff in the sterile operating room.

LIVING WILLS AND LEGAL DOCUMENTS

Untoward events are never planned or expected with medical or surgical procedures, and most of us do not want to even entertain this possibility. However, prior to your surgery date, the responsible thing to do is to set up certain legal documents that express your wishes in the event that you become unconscious or do not survive the surgery. These documents can provide peace of mind knowing that your wishes will be honored at all times. The following are optional legal documents, prepared in advance, that you can provide at the time you register.

- *Living Will:* Specifies what type of medical treatment, medication and resuscitation you want in the event you are unable to communicate your desires.

- *Health Care Proxy:* Designates another individual to make healthcare decisions if you are incapable of doing so.

- *Durable Power of Attorney:* Designates another individual to make financial decisions or transactions on your behalf if you become medically incapacitated.

TIPS FOR RECOVERY

- Clean your home thoroughly prior to surgery; you will not be able to for at least two to three weeks following your operation. Recruit family or friends to help post-op, or consider hiring a housekeeper.

- Buy thick sanitary pads to help absorb fluid from drain sites.

- Plan to wear comfortable, loose clothing initially after surgery.

- Place a bell and telephone with a speaker phone on your nightstand to request help.

- Have entertainment, such as books or a TV with a remote, readily available.

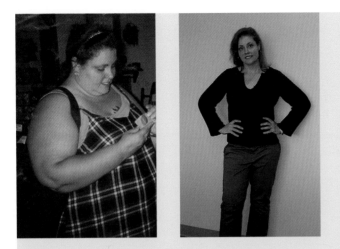

Patient Profile

Name:	Sally
Age:	43
Type of WL surgery:	Roux-en-Y Gastric Bypass
Amount of weight lost:	about 150 lbs
Original Weight:	298 lbs
Current Weight:	155 pounds

How long did it take you to lose the weight after surgery? About 18 months.

What has changed in your life after losing weight? I am able to be really active and participate in yoga, cross-country skiing, and dragonboat racing. I could never have considered these activities when I was overweight. My health has improved immensely. My blood pressure is normal. My GERD and asthma are gone. My arthritis hardly bothers me at all anymore. I had a good bit of self-confidence prior to losing weight, but I feel even more confident now that I don't feel self-conscious about my size. Basically, I feel like I got my life back, the life stolen by the excess pounds I was dragging around.

Which body contouring procedures have you had? Body lift procedure with inner thigh lift.

What was most frustrating about the excess skin after the weight loss? I worked very hard exercising to tone and shape my body, but you couldn't see the results because of all the ugly, wrinkled skin hanging on my body. It was difficult to see myself as successful in my weight loss when I was still wearing my size 26 skin on my much smaller body. I never wanted to look in the mirror when I was heavy because it was too painful to face the reality, but even after I lost the weight it was still painful to do. I looked deformed.

How has your life changed after the body contouring procedures? I have more body confidence and have a blast shopping for clothes. I no longer have to choose things based on how well they'll hide the hanging skin on my lower body. I even bought my first bikini!

What is your advice to others, contemplating body contouring? It is expensive, I know, but it is worth every penny. Getting rid of the excess skin is an important stage of the weight-loss journey and will make you feel much more confident about your body.

CHAPTER
5

Your Surgical Procedure:
What to Expect

When the day you have so carefully planned for and eagerly anticipated finally arrives —the day of your surgery—you can expect to feel a range of emotions, from excitement to nervousness to a bit of apprehension. Be assured, all of these feelings are normal. It's also reassuring to know that your plastic surgeon and the staff working with him or her understand these feelings and will do everything necessary to keep you safe and ensure the best possible result. Being well-informed and able to anticipate the day's events will also help alleviate your anxiety. You can look forward to a dramatic improvement in your body shape by the end of the day, as you begin your road to recovery.

WHAT TO WEAR

Wear comfortable, loose-fitting clothes —items you can easily put back on after surgery and that you do not have to pull over your head. Sweatpants, a baggy button-down shirt, a bathrobe, and slip-on shoes or slippers are good choices.

Do not wear jewelry to the surgery center. This includes earrings, rings, bracelets, necklaces, anklets, hairpins, and body-piercing rings. Most people think this is to guard against possible theft; however, the main reason is that *electrocautery*, a surgical instrument that uses a small electric current, is used to stop bleeding and jewelry can potentially conduct this current, posing a shock risk to you.

You cannot wear contact lenses, glasses, removable dental work, or wigs during your surgery. You may wish to leave them at home or put them in a safe place at the surgery center.

WHAT TO TAKE WITH YOU

Take a complete list of your medications, but do not take any medications with you unless your physician instructs you to do so. Although basic commodities are typically provided, you may want to take a small travel bag with your own toothbrush, nonelectrical shaving equipment, and any other personal items you use every day. Leave unnecessary valuables at home.

39

ARRIVING AT THE SURGERY CENTER

Your procedure will be performed at one of several locations: your doctor's surgical center, an independent outpatient ambulatory surgery center (ASC), or a hospital operating room. Days prior to your surgery, you will receive a telephone call from the surgeon's office telling you where the surgery will be performed and at what time you need to arrive. Expect to arrive one to two hours before your scheduled surgery time.

Registration

Upon arrival at the surgery center, you will proceed to patient registration to fill out necessary paperwork, show a photo ID, and provide health insurance information. You will be asked to sign a Conditions and Consent for Treatment form. If you have not already done so, you will then be asked to pay any insurance copayments, deductibles, or out-of-pocket expenses. In many cases you can preregister by telephone or online, which will expedite the check-in process considerably.

Inpatient or Outpatient

Depending on your recovery needs following surgery and what you decided with your surgeon, you will be registered as an *inpatient* or as an *outpatient*. As an inpatient, you will be admitted to the hospital with plans to stay in the hospital more than twenty-three hours for recovery. As an outpatient, also called an *ambulatory surgery patient*, you will be admitted to the *ambulatory surgery unit* (ASU) in the hospital or surgery center, where you are observed and discharged after surgery. This may be within a few hours after surgery or, in some cases, early the next morning after an overnight stay. In some cases, following discharge, you are transported to an overnight or extended care facility where you are observed by a licensed nurse or an aide.

Preoperative

After you have registered with the administrative offices, you'll most likely be met by a nurse or an aide who will escort you to a surgical waiting area. You will be given a gown to change into; you'll also be given a bag in which to store your clothes and other personal belongings. If necessary for your procedure, a nurse or medical assistant will tie back your hair with bands or clips. A cap may be placed on your head.

A nurse will drape you with a sheet or blanket to keep you warm. The nurse will then take your vital signs and perform a checklist, including a review of your medical history, medications you take, and allergies to drugs, foods, tape, latex, or iodine. At this point you will want to tell a member of the staff if you have any joint problems or replacements. Sharing this information will ensure the safest and most comfortable positioning during surgery.

You will then be asked to sign a consent form for the surgical procedure, which may be in addition to the form your surgeon had you sign in the office. You will also be asked to sign a blood transfusion consent form. This form reviews the risk of undergoing a blood transfusion and allows you to accept or decline a transfusion in the event that one is deemed necessary.

At this time, the nurse will probably insert an *intravenous line (IV)* into a vein in your arm or in the top of your hand. Anesthetic drugs will be administered through this line during your procedure. You'll also receive other medications such as narcotics for pain control, muscle relaxants, and perhaps steroids to help reduce postoperative swelling. At this point, you may also be given a sedative to help you relax. By the time you are taken into the operating room you will feel drowsy.

Just prior to surgery, the surgeon will place surgical markings on your body or reinforce the markings that were previously made. In the privacy of your waiting area, you may need to stand up and disrobe—partially or completely—so that these markings can be made. Wear your preferred undergarments so that he or she can place the skin markings in a way that ensures scars are kept within these boundaries. This is also a time to address any last minute questions.

IN THE OPERATING ROOM

As you enter the operating suite, you will notice several draped tables and stands holding numerous trays with instruments. This is the sterile field, which is free from bacteria or contamination. The scrub nurse will already be gowned and is likely to be in the process of setting up instruments and supplies.

A required "time-out" procedure will be conducted by the *circulating nurse*. To eliminate any chance of error, the surgical staff will verify your identity, the procedure, and body site to be operated on prior to the start of surgery.

Monitoring Devices

Once you have been transferred to a well-padded operating table, a number of monitoring devices will be attached to your body by the anesthesiologist. Adhesive electrodes are placed on your chest and extremities for continuous recording of your heart rhythm. A pulse oximeter clip-on or adhesive probe is attached to one of your fingers or your earlobe to measure oxygen saturation in your blood as well as your pulse rate. A blood pressure cuff is placed around your arm to measure blood pressure; you may feel temporary pressure in your arm as it inflates. A nerve stimulator may be applied, which causes muscle twitching, indicating the degree of muscle relaxation.

Temperature Control

You may find the room temperature to be on the cool or chilly side. This is in large part to allow members of the sterile operating team to work efficiently; they will be wearing gowns prone to heat retention. However, a primary concern throughout the procedure will be maintaining your core body temperature, and procedures will be in place both to monitor and to maintain it. To begin with, you will be covered with warm blankets as you enter the room. Additionally, a warming pad may be placed on the table beneath your body. Fluids that are administered to you can be warmed. Also, your body will be mostly covered with sterile drapes during surgery, exposing only the operative site to heat loss. Frequently, a forced air heating blanket will be applied to your upper or lower body.

Preventing Blood Clot Formation

Prior to receiving anesthesia, you will likely have a soft compression sleeve wrapped around your legs or your feet, especially if you are receiving general anesthesia or undergoing a long operation.

This device, technically known as a *sequential compression device* (SCD), inflates and tightens much like a blood pressure cuff and is intended to prevent the formation of blood clots in the legs. Such clots, known as deep vein thrombosis, or DVT, can break off and obstruct the lungs, called a pulmonary embolism, or PE, which can be a life-threatening condition.

After surgery, you will continue to wear these compression sleeves while in bed and until you are walking. In fact, your surgeon will want you up and walking as quickly as possible, frequently by the first day after the surgery. Getting out of bed and walking is one of the most important ways to reduce the risk of DVT and PE. Other precautions that are sometimes also taken to reduce blood clot formation include injections of blood thinners such as heparin.

There is still a chance for DVT and PE during your recovery at home, but this risk gradually decreases over a couple of months. You can greatly minimize this risk by walking at least three times a day, avoiding prolonged sitting in one position as may occur during a long car ride, and staying well hydrated by drinking at least eight glasses of water a day.

Administration of Anesthesia

An anesthesiologist or certified registered nurse anesthetist (CRNA) will deliver your anesthesia. If you are having general anesthesia, the anesthesiologist will begin by having you breathe 100 percent oxygen using a face mask. You will be asked to take slow deep breaths. Within minutes you will fall asleep. At this point, the breathing tube is carefully inserted by the anesthesiol-ogist and secured in place. There are several types of anesthesia.

General Anesthesia

For most major or extensive body contouring procedures you will receive *general anesthesia*, which places you in a deep sleep or essentially unconscious during surgery. During general anesthesia you will not be able to feel pain in your body. Your anesthesiologist has control over your breathing and you are comfortable during lengthy procedures. Medication is usually administered through your intravenous line or by inhalation of an anesthetic gas.

This type of anesthesia requires a plastic tube to be placed in your mouth to control air movement through your windpipe, or *trachea*; this assists in your breathing as well as in the administration of oxygen and anesthetic gas. This tube can be either a laryngeal mask airway (LMA) or an endotracheal tube (ETT). Complete muscle relaxation or paralysis, which may be necessary with abdominal procedures, is possible only with a general anesthetic.

Regional Anesthesia

With *regional anesthesia*, only a portion of the body is numbed—this is done by injecting anesthetic near the nerves that supply sensation to the area of the body where surgery is to be performed. For example, it may numb only the lower half of your body. This does not alter your level of consciousness.

The most common type of regional anesthesia for body contouring is an epidural or spinal. In this case, anesthetic is carefully injected into your back, near the nerves that exit from the spinal cord as they fan out to supply sensation. This is ordinarily done in the operating room, where you will either be bent forward in a sitting position or lying on your side in the fetal position. In either case, producing curvature in your back is important in placing the epidural or spinal. The medication is injected such that the surgical site falls within the boundaries of the area that is numbed. With an epidural, a small catheter can be left in place for continuous or prolonged administration of anesthetic, sometimes for one to two days following surgery. One potential benefit is that you are able to move around sooner and more easily following surgery because of this targeted pain control.

Local Anesthesia

This type of anesthesia refers to the injection of a *local anesthetic*, drugs that deaden the sensation of pain in a specific area without putting you to sleep. These injections are similar to those you might receive at your dentist. For body contouring surgery, local anesthetics can provide pain control during and after surgery. Local anesthetic is often injected in combination with saline and adrenaline (epinephrine) in a mixture called a *wetting solution*, particularly during liposuction. The addition of epinephrine allows for the safe use of greater doses of local anesthetic and also helps reduce blood loss.

Monitored Anesthesia Care (MAC)

Monitored anesthesia involves intravenous sedation and produces a twilight sleep. Most often, MAC is combined with local or regional anesthesia. Since recovery from MAC is typically more rapid compared to general anesthesia, many plastic surgeons prefer to use MAC with a local for a number of their procedures.

Insertion of a Urinary Catheter

If your surgery is to last longer than three to four hours, it is likely that a Foley catheter will be inserted. This tube runs up through the urethra and into the bladder; this helps keep track of fluid balance and will keep the bladder empty during surgery. Sometimes, the catheter is removed in the operating room at the close of your operation. Otherwise, it is easily removed the day following surgery. You should experience no pain once the catheter is inside the bladder, although on occasion you may have the urge to urinate even though your bladder is empty.

The Skin Prep

Your skin is cleansed and decontaminated with a chemical disinfecting agent, typically Betadine (povidone-iodine). If you have an allergy to iodine, another agent such as chlorhexidine will be used.

Your body is then covered with sterile surgical drapes. The only part of your body left exposed will be the part where surgery is to be performed. The drapes are intended to minimize the transfer of bacteria to the surgical site.

UNDERGOING THE SURGERY

Before making the first incision, the surgeon will likely inject local anesthetic containing epinephrine into the tissues and along the incision lines. This causes vasoconstriction (narrowing) of small blood vessels, resulting in less blood loss when the incision is made. The surgeon will then make an incision, using the markings that were previously placed on your skin as a guide, since your tissues will shift and take on a much different position when you are lying flat on the operating table.

Removal of Tissue Excess

Tissue excess following weight loss is primarily comprised of skin. This is treated by direct excision of skin, which will also include the *subcutaneous* or fatty layer beneath the skin. Additional pockets of *fatty tissue* may be removed with liposuction. Commonly, the weight of tissue removed ranges from ten to fifteen pounds or more. What happens to this tissue? Most of the time it is discarded as medical waste. However, there are instances when tissue is sent to pathology for examination. Such may be the case with breast tissue excised during a breast reduction to ensure that there are no changes associated with breast cancer.

Liposuction

Liposuction (*suction-assisted lipectomy* or *lipoplasty*) refers to the use of a vacuum to create suction through a small hollow metal tube or *cannula*. When passed back and forth through the *subcutaneous layer* fatty deposits are removed.

The development of liposuction revolutionized body contouring surgery, and it is one of the most commonly performed procedures. However, it is important to understand that liposuction primarily treats fat and not skin. It has less of a role when there is damage to the skin with loss of tone or if there is skin excess. In this situation, using liposuction as the only form of treatment will worsen deformity due to problems related primarily to the skin. Only youthful and elastic skin has the ability to retract and conform to the underlying contour when fat is removed.

However, following massive weight loss, liposuction does serve as an important tool for your plastic surgeon to help shape your body by removing stubborn fat deposits that do not go away with diet or exercise.

There are specialized forms of liposuction, including ultrasound-assisted liposuction (UAL). During UAL, ultrasonic energy is first used to melt the fat, making it easier to remove with suction. UAL is particularly beneficial in very fibrous or dense areas, such as is commonly found on the back or in the male breast. Power-assisted liposuction (PAL) refers to a suction cannula that automatically moves back and forth, also making it easier to pass through denser tissues and also resulting in less fatigue for the surgeon during extensive procedures.

Restoring Deep Tissues

Cellular structures deep under the skin also develop laxity with time and contribute to changes in your body contour. These structures must be tightened to restore your contour. This may be achieved by tightening the abdominal muscle during an abdominoplasty procedure or the muscle in the neck during a neck lift.

Hemostasis

Controlling blood loss from the incision sites is referred to as obtaining *hemostasis*. Many patients ask whether they will have much blood loss. The amount lost depends on how much tissue needs to be excised.

Although your body is very effective at controlling blood loss through natural clotting mechanisms, meticulous surgical technique will also used; this includes the use of electrocautery, which stops bleeding by coagulating small blood vessels with an electrical current. Larger blood vessels are tied with sutures. As mentioned, epinephrine injected at surgical sites also greatly reduces blood loss by constricting blood vessels. In some cases, your surgeon may use a biological tissue glue made with clotting factors, called *fibrin glue*, to seal the wound and stop minor bleeding.

In most cases, the blood loss is very tolerable, and new blood cells will be produced in your bone marrow as you recover over a period of a couple of months. Although transfusions are rarely required, this chance does increase when anemia is already present and with extensive and prolonged surgeries.

Insertion of Drains

In many cases, your plastic surgeon will need to insert one or more small drainage tubes to prevent fluid buildup at the surgical site. A soft tube will be placed under the skin through a tiny opening near the main incision. This drainage tube is then attached to a small suction bulb and is referred to as a *closed suction drain.*

Why does fluid collect, making these drains necessary? The process of tightening the skin requires separating it from the underlying tissue structures to allow it to move freely, not unlike having to lift a bed sheet, then pulling it down over the mattress for a smoother fit. This is called *undermining*, and it disrupts blood vessels between the skin and the deeper tissues. The greater the amount of undermining, the higher the likelihood of serum accumulation exceeding what your body can naturally absorb; this leads to a collection of fluid under the skin called a seroma. In situations where liposuction has been extensive, this

fluid collection can also occur. A seroma may prevent proper wound healing; in some cases, the fluid becomes infected. So, until the wound surfaces seal together adequately, drains provide an important safety valve. You may be asked to take an antibiotic to minimize the chance for infection.

The number of drains required depends on the size of the incision. Larger procedures require more drains. For example, an abdominoplasty may require two to three drains, whereas a body lift may require four to six drains.

The length of time a drain needs to stay in place depends on the quantity of fluid that is draining. The collection bulb for a drain is secured to your clothing and readily concealed. You will be taught how to care for the drains at home. This includes maintaining a daily record of the quantity of fluid collected.

There will be a gradual decrease in the amount that drains, as well as a gradual change from red to pink and finally to a straw-colored fluid. These changes determine when your surgeon removes the drains, a quick procedure in the office with minimal to no discomfort. Drains that you may have had with prior weight loss surgery or with other intra-abdominal procedures are usually more uncomfortable or painful when removed. Some drains, particularly those used for an abdominoplasty procedure, stay in place for two to three weeks if the output is high. Others, such as those used for a face lift, are usually removed within 24 hours.

Not every body contouring procedure requires a drain. For example, they are not necessary in most breast procedures. In some situations, your surgeon may be able to use a biological tissue glue to seal the wound surfaces, eliminating the need for a drain.

Closing the Incisions

The final surgical step involves closing or suturing the incisions. In body contouring procedures, surgeons usually perform multiple layers of suturing to adequately close layers of tissue. In some cases, there can be as many as five separate levels of suturing.

The type of suture used is largely determined by your surgeon's preference. To provide a greater degree of long-term support, he or she may place permanent sutures in the deepest layers of tissue, where you will not be able to see them. Sutures that are absorbable are placed closer to the surface of the skin; these sutures typically dissolve over a period of weeks to months while the incision is healing and the skin is regaining its strength.

In many cases, there are no visible sutures or staples at the surface of the skin and none that require removal. Any sutures that are visible at the surface are typically removed in the office within a three- to ten-day period. Normally, adhesive strips of tape, called Steri-strips, are applied to the incision to provide extra support. In some cases, your surgeon may instead apply a liquid skin adhesive called Dermabond. This strengthens the skin closure at the surface and also provides a barrier to bacteria, water, and other contaminants. Normally, this clear barrier begins to peel off and can be removed within a couple of weeks.

Dressing Placement

Gauze dressing is applied to the incision when the closure is completed. This helps to protect the incision as well as to absorb any drainage, which is normal in the first twenty-four to forty-eight hours. You may also be placed in a supportive garment, such as an elastic binder placed around your waist following an abdominoplasty procedure. In some cases, it will be an elastic garment that you were fitted for prior to surgery.

Awakening from Anesthesia

While the dressings are being placed, you will be awakened from anesthesia. The anesthesiologist will give you adequate pain medication to ensure that you are comfortable as you regain consciousness. He or she will ask you to open your eyes and to take deep breaths. When you are breathing adequately, the breathing tube will be removed and oxygen will be administered through a mask. With the dressings in place, the operating room staff will then carefully transfer you to a hospital bed.

Length of Surgery

How long will you be in surgery? Of course, this depends on the type of procedure or combination of procedures you are having and the severity of your skin excess. There are other factors, including your surgeon's technique and whether another surgeon is involved.

Of the total length of time spent in the operating room, a significant portion can be spent on procedures other than surgery. For example, it will take some time to put you to sleep as well as to allow you to wake up at the end of surgery. Another time-consuming aspect of body contouring

Length of Surgeries
National Averages

Procedure	Length (hours)
Abdominoplasty (tummy tuck)	2 – 5
Body Lift	Up to 8
Breast Lift	1.5 – 3.5
Breast Reduction	2 – 4
Buttock Lift	2
Thigh Lift	2
Upper Arm Lift	2
Face lift	2 – 3

From American Society for Aesthetic Plastic Surgery (ASAPS) Database, 2004

surgery is positioning. This refers to the process of positioning your body on the operating room table to provide for the best possible exposure of the surgical site, while ensuring your comfort and safety. Especially when multiple areas of your body are to be addressed, a significant amount of time can be spent carefully positioning and repositioning during the procedure.

During a lengthy operation, your surgeon will periodically provide an update regarding your progress to family and/or friends in the waiting room.

POSTOPERATIVE

The Recovery Room

From the operating room you will be taken to the recovery room, also known as the *postoperative anesthesia care unit* (PACU). Here, you will continue to be under the care of the anesthesiologist as well as a certified nurse. You'll probably stay in the PACU for about one hour, providing for a smooth emergence from anesthesia.

As you emerge from anesthesia, you will begin to feel tightness at your incision site. It is best that you ask the nursing staff for help with initial movements such as turning, and that you provide some feedback regarding the level of tightness, to prevent disruption of any suture lines. In the PACU, you will remain attached to monitoring devices. In addition to checking your level of consciousness, the recovery room nurse will examine your dressings and drains regularly for any problems.

From the PACU, you will be transported to a hospital room if you are an inpatient or to the ambulatory surgery unit if you are an outpatient. Unless you are scheduled for an overnight twenty-three-hour stay, you will be discharged to the care of a responsible adult for transfer back to your home or to a nearby overnight care facility.

SIDE EFFECTS OF SURGERY

Chills

Many patients feel cold and shiver immediately after waking up from surgery. There are several reasons for this. During some operations in which larger sections of the skin's surface are open, there can be significant loss of body heat. Also, the anesthesia may affect the hypothalamus in the brain, which is the body's thermostat. As the anesthetic agent dissipates in your bloodstream, you'll feel warmer. You will be covered with a warming blanket if your body temperature is low. Sometimes, you will also be administered medication to control severe shivering.

Types of Scars

- **Immature:** A new or young scar. Typically feels hard, thick and raised. Has red or purple coloration.
- **Mature:** The final form of a scar when the remodeling process is complete. Typically flat, soft and white.
- **Hypertrophic:** An abnormal scar that is thick and raised.
- **Keloid:** An abnormal scar that grows to extend beyond the boundaries of the initial scar.

Pain and Nausea

You will be assessed frequently for pain and nausea. Often, you will have been given preemptive doses of strong anti-nausea and pain medication prior to even leaving the operating room. Additional dosing will be ordered by the anesthesiologist in the PACU as required.

Dry Mouth

Dry mouth is very common immediately after surgery. It is best quenched with ice chips at first, especially if you have any degree of nausea.

Irritated Throat or Nasal Passages

You may find that your throat is sore, or you may be hoarse as the result of the breathing tube used during surgery. The soreness should disappear within twenty-four to forty-eight hours. In the meantime, drinking fluids or sucking on a throat lozenge may bring relief.

YOUR HOSPITAL STAY

Your surgeon will write specific orders for your hospital postoperative care.

Depending on the extent of surgery, you may be in the hospital from one to four days, but rarely longer.

Getting out of Bed

If you stay overnight in the hospital, your surgeon will want you out of bed and moving as soon as possible. Typically, this is no later than the first morning after surgery. This is to prevent the formation of blood clots in the legs. At first, moving will be a slow and tedious process, requiring assistance from the nursing staff, who will be aware of any activity restrictions. Often, your surgeon will have ordered a trapeze (metal frame) to be attached to your bed, which will help greatly with transfers into and out of bed. While you are in bed, the sequential compression devices (SCDs) will be kept on your legs as an additional precaution against blood clot formation.

Diet

After surgery, you will usually be started on a clear liquid diet. A limiting factor may be nausea resulting from anesthesia or strong pain medication. These conditions typically resolve within twenty-four hours as the anesthetic drugs leave your body. Until you are capable of drinking an adequate amount, you will be administered intravenous saline solution to replace fluid losses from surgery and to keep you hydrated. Even when you are back at home, it is best to stick with a bland diet for the first few days.

Deep-Breathing Exercises

You will be instructed on the use of an incentive spirometer, a plastic device that promotes deep breathing. This will assist in keeping your lungs fully expanded, preventing the development of *pulmonary atelectasis*, incomplete expansion of the lung, which can cause fever and increases the risk for pneumonia.

Sleep Apnea

If you suffer from obstructive sleep apnea and use a *continuous positive airway pressure* (CPAP) machine or similar device at home, it is important to let your surgeon know this in advance. The hospital respiratory therapist will provide for postoperative therapy, and in some cases you may want to bring your own device from home.

Regular Monitoring

The nursing staff will check your temperature, blood pressure, and pulse on a regular basis. They will also monitor your fluid intake and output, including that of any drains. Your surgeon will monitor your daily progress and look for any problems related to surgery.

ADDITIONAL SIDE EFFECTS OF SURGERY

As you continue to recover, you will experience the normal side effects of surgery. The following is a list of symptoms to be anticipated after body contouring surgery. As these changes are an expected result of surgery and part of your recovery, they are not considered complications unless they persist, prolong recovery, or otherwise impact your final result.

Swelling and Bruising

The swelling from surgery will peak at seventy-two hours. Thereafter, it will subside significantly over the next couple of weeks. However, although 75 percent of

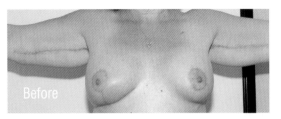

Two months after an extended arm lift and breast lift procedure. Scars are immature.

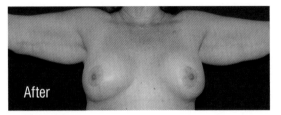

One year after an extended arm lift and breast lift surgery. Scars are now mature.

swelling may have subsided within six weeks, it may take six months to two years for complete resolution. Bruising may develop around incision sites or in lower areas of the body where gravity directs the blood. Bruising will resolve at a faster rate than swelling, typically undergoing a number of color changes until completely gone within two to three weeks.

Soreness and Discomfort

This is usually mild to moderate pain which should improve with time. Take prescription pain medication regularly, at least early on in the recovery period, to provide adequate pain relief and prevent sudden spikes.

Numbness

Some nerves will be affected during surgery. This may cause temporary numbness; normal sensation usually returns within three to four months, although areas of permanent numbness can occur. You may experience itching or shooting sensations as the nerve endings recover.

Scars

Scars go through a maturation process. At first, they may feel thick and hard. A new or immature scar is raised and has pink, red or purple coloration. As time progresses, the scar will feel softer, become flat, and the color will fade to your normal skin color. This process, however, will take at least six months and up to one to two years to complete. Importantly, although scars will fade with time, they are, nevertheless, permanent. Some individuals, in particular those with darker skin, may be prone to forming abnormal scars, such as hypertrophic or keloid scars, which are more noticeable and can cause burning and itching. Your plastic surgeon will review this risk and potential treatment strategies.

Feeling Depressed

Feelings of depression are normal and temporary for the first few weeks following surgery. You may even feel a period of let-down or question your decision to have had surgery. This is a natural phase, and as your body heals you will also feel better emotionally. Remind yourself that it will take some time to see the final results of surgery. Although support from family and friends can be helpful, they may not completely understand what a normal recovery involves. Your surgeon and his or her staff will honestly inform you of your progress based on their knowledge and experience. If feelings of anxiety or depression are severe or persist beyond three to four weeks, professional evaluation may be advised by your surgeon.

DISCHARGE FROM THE HOSPITAL

Your surgeon will determine when you are ready for discharge. Important criteria for discharge include being able to maintain an adequate level of pain control, the ability to drink an adequate amount to stay hydrated, and no evidence of fever or other serious complications. Additionally, it's important to have a responsible adult available to drive you home.

Before you leave, the nursing staff will review postoperative instructions with you and teach wound and surgical drain care. You may be given medications to take home with you or a prescription for medication to have filled. In many cases, you will have filled these prescriptions prior to your surgery.

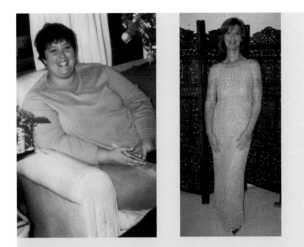

Patient Profile

Name: Heather
Age: 35
Type of WL surgery: Banded Gastric Bypass
Original Weight: 385 pounds
Amount of weight lost: 250 pounds
Current Weight: 157 pounds

How long did it take you to lose the weight after surgery? Approximately 18 months.

What has changed in your life after losing weight? There have been many changes. I have divorced and plan to remarry; I have moved and changed jobs. I feel a great new confidence when I encounter the challenges of my life now. It is wonderful to be able to work each day and not be exhausted at the end of the day. I look back at my life before and realize why I was tired. Each day I carried the equivalent of a football player on my back.

Which body contouring procedures have you had? Arm lift, breast lift, and body lift.

What was most frustrating about the excess skin after the weight loss? It has been difficult learning new strategies for dealing with the fears, frustrations and challenges of my new life, because my previous strategy of using food is no longer an option. Also, I can no longer blame being fat if I fail at something or encounter a difficulty.

How has your life changed after the body contouring procedures? I am a much happier person. I feel a lot more confident about trying on clothes. And, I can be more active now. Before, I always had to offer excuses for not joining various activities. I feel more comfortable being in public now that I have had excess skin removed. After all a fat person is just a fat person, but with the excess skin people wonder who is this Shar-pei-looking person and what happened to her?

What is your advice to others, contemplating body contouring? Work out a payment plan and do it! You and your quality of life are worth it. You deserve it and all the happiness of life, no matter what your insurance company says.

CHAPTER 6

Post-Surgical Pain Management

How much will it hurt? How long will it hurt? Will I be able to handle the pain? These are likely some of the biggest concerns you have going into any surgery.

It's true that, with few exceptions, most contouring surgeries involve some pain. However, the amount and the quality of pain will differ, depending on the type of surgery and the individual. Some people experience little or no pain while others report a significant amount of pain or discomfort. However, even for the most extensive of procedures, postoperative pain is easily controlled and very tolerable for most people. For everyone involved in your care, pain control will be a top priority in the immediate postoperative period and as you continue to heal.

TYPES OF PAIN

Based on location, pain receptor activation will cause three primary types of pain: *somatic, visceral,* and *neuropathic.* In general, if you have had weight loss surgery, you probably experienced the visceral type pain that is characteristically deep and crampy with pressure-like or squeezing qualities. It is poorly localized and related to internal organs.

Visceral pain is quite different in quality from the pain following most body contouring procedures, which is largely of the somatic type. Somatic pain has a dull and throbbing quality; occasionally it can be sharper and prickling. This pain is typically well localized to the skin and underlying soft tissues. An example is the pain from an incision. In fact, if you had laparoscopic weight loss surgery with very small skin incisions, the amount of this type of pain may have been little to none compared to pain from a body contouring procedure, such as the body lift, where the incision is extensive.

The third type of pain, neuropathic pain, has a severe shooting and burning quality, which is related to nerve injury. An example is sciatica from a pinched nerve in the back, with pain radiating down the leg.

Often, you may experience overlap of these different pain types. In addition, there are other factors that contribute to pain or discomfort, including the side effects of anesthesia.

PAIN AFTER BODY CONTOURING SURGERY

The procedures that typically require the greatest amount of postoperative pain

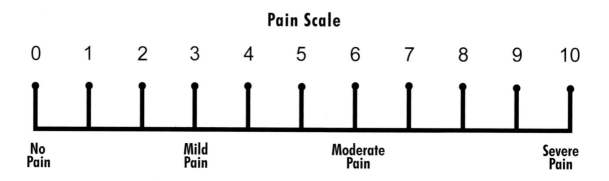

Pain Scale

| 0 | 1 | 2 | 3 | 4 | 5 | 6 | 7 | 8 | 9 | 10 |

No Pain   Mild Pain   Moderate Pain   Severe Pain

control are those involving the torso or midsection of your body. These procedures include the abdominoplasty and body lift, which require long incisions and often involve significant tightening of deep tissues such as the abdominal muscles. Routine movements such as getting out of bed or standing up from a chair require the use of these abdominal muscles, which may further aggravate your pain or discomfort.

For a procedure such as the body lift, one of the primary reasons to keep you in the hospital at least one night and often longer is to ensure adequate pain control. You can expect moderate postoperative pain which subsides significantly over twenty-four to forty-eight hours. Mild to moderate pain is then readily controlled with prescription pain pills. At ten to fourteen days you will be able to transition to non-prescription pain pills for mild pain symptoms, with an occasional need for stronger prescription pain pills. By two to three weeks only rarely will you require pain medication. By six to eight weeks, there may be mild occasional discomfort as you are allowed to begin more strenuous activity. For most outpatient surgeries, this time frame is compressed. Pain following these procedures is typically mild to

moderate and easily controlled with prescription pain pills.

ASSESSING PAIN

You will be assessed for postoperative pain, including objective quantification. There are various pain rating scales, the most common of which has you rate your level of pain on a scale of one to ten, with ten being the worst pain you have ever experienced. To be comfortable, your pain should be kept at a rating of three or less. It is important for you to openly communicate your needs to allow for proper assessment and successful management of your pain

METHODS OF PAIN MANAGEMENT

Postoperative pain control begins in the operating room. This may be done by placing an epidural catheter that is kept in place for postoperative pain management or through the injection of local anesthetic that continues to work for some time after surgery. As you awaken in the operating room, you will also be administered adequate pain medication intravenously to keep you comfortable and prevent you from experiencing intense pain. For continued pain management there are a number of options utilizing modern medicines and effective delivery methods.

Postoperatively, your doctor will write orders for the administration of pain medication. There are various administration routes for most pain medications, including oral (pill or liquid), rectal suppository, sublingual (placed below the tongue), transdermal (skin patch), neuraxial (epidural or spinal), or injections, which may be intravenous, subcutaneous, or intramuscular. The intravenous and oral methods tend to be used most frequently.

Opioid Medications

Commonly referred to as *narcotics*, drugs that dull pain and make you very drowsy, *opioids* are highly effective against moderate to severe postoperative pain and are the mainstay of therapy. They work by blocking special pain receptors in the central nervous system, called opioid receptors, preventing delivery of the message of pain. Commonly used narcotics include morphine, meperidine (Demerol), hydromorphone (Dilaudid), and fentanyl. The most frequently prescribed pain medications that you will go home with are also opioids, such as Vicodin or Tylenol with codeine.

Although very effective at pain relief, opioids can have significant side effects, including sedation, depressed or slowed breathing, nausea and vomiting, confusion or delirium, low blood pressure, itching, and constipation. Often your physician may need to give you additional medications to relieve such side effects.

Nonopioid Medications

Nonsteroidal Anti-inflammatory Drugs (NSAIDs), are nonnarcotic and good for treating mild to moderate pain. They work by blocking the production of substances in the body that cause pain and inflammation. Although they are not as strong as opioids, they do not cause as many side effects and are nonsedating. They also have an anti-inflammatory action, which can control pain by reducing irritation directly at the surgical site. The most potent of the prescription NSAIDs, ketorolac (Toradol), is often given for moderate postoperative pain and can help reduce the amount of narcotic medication and associated side effects. Common over-the-counter NSAIDs include aspirin, Motrin, Advil and Aleve.

Conditions that can limit or prevent exposure to NSAIDs include stomach ulcer disease, high blood pressure, cardiovascular disease, and kidney or platelet dysfunction. If you have had gastric bypass surgery, you will want to get clearance from your bariatric surgeon prior to any extensive use of these drugs, since your stomach pouch is more prone to ulcer formation.

Another over-the-counter medication, acetaminophen, or Tylenol works by elevating your pain threshold and is effective for relieving mild pain. It is also a good fever reducer. It does not have the same side effects as the NSAIDs and is safer to use if you have a stomach ulcer, high blood pressure, or kidney disease. Also, it will not cause bleeding problems like the NSAIDs. However, it can cause severe liver damage, especially if there is existing liver disease. Importantly, there are a number of medications that contain Tylenol, such as Vicodin, and you need to pay close attention not to exceed the maximum recommended dose in a twenty-four-hour period.

Patient-Controlled Analgesia (PCA)

Patient-controlled analgesia (PCA) is a form of pain management that allows you to administer your own pain relief. The pain medication, which is usually an opioid, is delivered through an intravenous or an epidural line, which is attached to a pump. By pressing a button, your can administer a predetermined dose of a pain medication when needed. The pump may also be programmed to administer a continuous dose. To safeguard against overdosing, the pump is programmed with a limit as to how much of the drug may be given in a specified time period. On the downside, PCA may lead to a greater level of sedation and delayed ability to move around effectively. Nevertheless, PCA is widely used in the United States because it works well and has a good safety record.

Pain Relief Ball

At the end of the operation, your surgeon may implant a small catheter into the incision site for continuous infusion of local anesthetic after surgery. This catheter is attached to a small high-tech balloon, called a pain relief ball which is filled with local anesthetic. This system can infuse local anesthetic directly into the surgical site for up to five days. This can cut down on the amount of narcotic medication and episodes of breakthrough pain.

IMPORTANCE OF CONTROLLING PAIN

The reason for controlling pain seems obvious—who wants to experience pain? However, there are other reasons why it is important to control the magnitude or intensity of pain during and after your surgery. Having pain under control means a faster recovery from surgery. Uncontrolled pain may weaken your body's immune system.

Furthermore, your experience with surgery will be a positive one when pain is properly controlled, decreasing the risk for complications. For example, pain that is tolerable allows you to walk sooner after surgery, which is important in preventing blood clot formation. On the other hand, if a significant amount of pain is preventing you from taking deep breaths, you are more prone to develop pneumonia. Inadequate pain control can lead to fear, anxiety, and depression, which in turn may worsen your pain. Although you may be concerned about forming an addiction, this risk is extremely low when strong pain medications are used for the purpose of controlling postoperative pain.

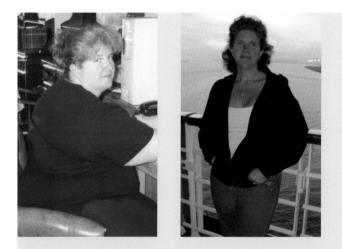

Patient Profile

Name: Rebecca

Age: 44

Type of WL surgery: Roux-en-Y Gastric Bypass

Amount of weight lost: 147 pounds

Original Weight: 325 pounds

Current Weight: 186 pounds

How long did it take you to lose the weight? Most of it in the first nine months. I had drastic loss in the first three months.

What has changed in your life after losing weight? I have greater self esteem. Better health. I have changed the way I think about food. My priorities in life have changed. Health and fitness have become a big part of my life.

Which body contouring procedures have you had to date? Abdominoplasty with an incisional hernia repair, breast lift with implants, and an arm lift.

What was most frustrating about the excess skin after the weight loss? My negative body image. I worked so hard to lose the weight, but then I had skin hanging. It was painful, especially when I would walk fast or jog. I also had irritation under the skin folds, which led to rashes and infections.

How has your life changed after the body contouring procedures? I feel free from my fat body of the past. I feel sexy and attractive—something I have never felt in my life. I have more self confidence in both my personal life and my professional life. I have a better quality of life. My favorite moment was when I put on a size 12 Levis jeans. I have never worn a size 12 in anything and never owned a pair of Levis jeans. It really made me feel like I had achieved my goal.

What is your advice to others, contemplating body contouring? Don't rush into the surgery right after your weight loss. Get your weight stabilized. Remember it may take a few surgeries to contour the areas that you feel need it.

CHAPTER 7

Abdomen and Waist Contouring

If you're like many people who've lost a significant amount of weight, one of your main complaints is the excess skin and fat that hangs from your abdomen. This is the area where the greatest deformity develops after massive weight loss. Although abdominal contouring surgery has been performed for over a century, modern surgical procedures now give plastic surgeons a number of options to choose from and greater ability to restore a sleeker contour to the abdomen and waistline following massive weight loss.

FULL ABDOMINOPLASTY

If massive weight loss has left you with excess skin on your abdomen, you probably will benefit most from a *full abdominoplasty*, the abdominal contouring procedure commonly referred to as a *tummy tuck*. This procedure, also called a standard abdominoplasty, has rapidly become popular for both men and women following significant weight reduction. It addresses several problems in the abdominal region—loose skin and fat as well as a relaxed underlying abdominal wall. Through a full abdominoplasty, your surgeon can remove excess skin and fat, contouring your abdomen from the pubic area to the breastbone.

Additionally, a full abdominoplasty includes tightening of the abdominal muscles, which is often necessary in shaping the abdomen. These muscles are wrapped in *fascia*, a supportive layer of tissue that lies beneath the fat. This fascia is prone to stretching from obesity or pregnancy, creating a condition called *rectus diastasis* in which the muscles separate. Some people are more likely to develop this condition than others. With diastasis, the stomach or abdomen bulges significantly, but this disappears when lying flat. Although diastasis does not represent a danger, moderate to severe cases can affect posture and even contribute to back pain. Often, the degree of muscle separation cannot be determined until the time of surgery.

As part of the tummy tuck procedure, liposuction may be used in a limited fashion to remove fat deposits in the upper abdomen and flanks, or "love handle" areas. You may benefit from more extensive abdominal liposuction when you are fully healed from your abdominoplasty procedure, a minimum of three months later.

UNDERGOING A FULL ABDOMINOPLASTY

To perform a full abdominoplasty, the surgeon makes a long "bikini-line" incision across the lower abdomen. It begins at the top of the pubic area and then slopes gently upward towards your hip bone. The incision is placed so it can be hidden by undergarments and swimwear. This incision generally runs from hip bone to hip bone. A lift of the pubic area is performed in cases where there is significant drooping.

A second circular incision is made to separate the navel or belly button from surrounding skin and fat. The navel "stalk," the part that is anchored to your abdominal wall, is not moved and remains attached at roughly the level of your hip bones. After the incisions are made, the abdominal skin and fat are carefully separated as an abdominal skin flap from the abdominal wall. By elevating the abdominal skin flap off the fascia, the plastic surgeon can work on either repairing a hernia or correcting diastasis.

The process of diastasis repair, or tightening of the abdominal muscles, is a procedure in which the fascia is tightened with sutures in the middle, usually from the breastbone down to the pubic bone. Called *fascial plication*, this procedure pulls the rectus muscles back together, similar to creating an internal corset, producing a flatter abdomen and more shapely waist. The amount of flattening or tightening may be limited by excess fat that remains on the inside of the abdomen.

Your surgeon may place a small removable catheter just below the fascia where the pain fibers are located to allow for infusion of local anesthetic after surgery.

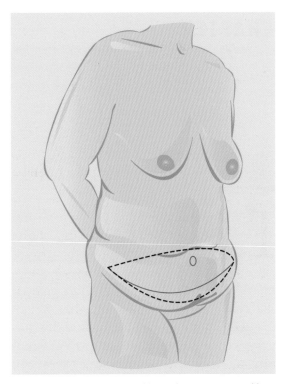

Standard abdominoplasty. Dotted line indicates incision. Red line indicates scar.

The abdominal skin flap is then pulled downward like a window shade and excess skin and fat are trimmed. At this point the operating table is adjusted to produce a slight bend at your waist, thereby allowing for resection of excess tissue. The surgeon then creates a hole in the abdominal skin flap at the level of the navel stalk. This hole becomes the new opening for your belly button, which is sewn to the abdominal skin flap. This leaves a circular scar around a smaller and shapelier belly button.

At this point, the surgeon will begin to close the incision, using several layers of sutures. Later, only a few sutures around the belly button will require removal. Typically, two or three drainage tubes are placed under the abdominal skin flap, and these are brought out through small openings in the pubic area, where they are secured with sutures.

The incisions are covered with gauze dressing, as are the drain sites. An elastic abdominal binder is placed around your waist for support and comfort. From the operating table you will be transferred to a bed, which is adjusted to keep you bent at the waist.

MODIFIED ABDOMINOPLASTY PROCEDURES

Your plastic surgeon may choose to use one of several modified versions of the standard abdominoplasty, some which have greater ability to address specific issues following massive weight loss. The scars may differ for each of these procedures.

Extended Abdominoplasty

This procedure can also remove the roll of loose skin and fat that wraps around the waistline or the love handle area. Of the abdominoplasty procedures, the extended procedure results in the longest scar, extending onto the back area.

Anchor (Fleur-de-lis) Abdominoplasty

This procedure has greater ability to tighten the abdomen above the level of the belly button when very large skin folds are present. It does, however, leave an additional vertical scar. This additional scar may not be a concern if there is already a scar present from a prior open bariatric procedure.

High-Lateral-Tension Abdominoplasty

During this procedure, the surgeon places greater emphasis on pulling the skin tighter at the outer waistline. The scar is otherwise the same as a standard abdominoplasty procedure scar. There is a slightly greater chance of "dog-ear" formation which may need later revision. What is a dog-ear? It's an area of excess

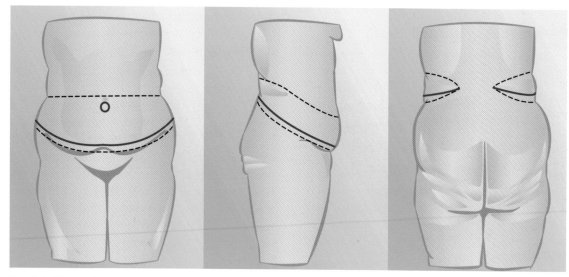

Extended abdominoplasty

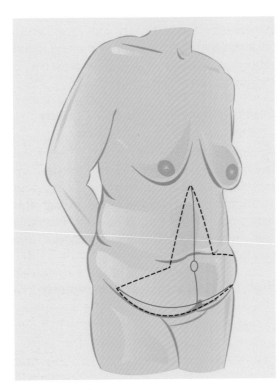

Anchor abdominoplasty

skin at the end of an incision that may protrude like a dog ear.

Reverse (Upper) Abdominoplasty

This procedure is done primarily to contour the upper abdomen when there is a significant amount of skin looseness present. By placing the incision in the crease below the breasts, the skin is pulled upward, opposite to a standard abdomin-oplasty. This procedure is well-suited for women who are having a breast lift or a reduction, where the same incision is used and the scar is hidden by the contour of the breasts. A standard abdominoplasty may still be necessary for contouring of the lower abdominal area.

Less Invasive Abdominal Contouring Procedures

The mini-abdominoplasty, also known as a partial or mini–tummy tuck, is performed by making a shorter incision along the bikini-line. The endoscopic abdominoplasty, on the other hand, is performed through small incisions and is done primarily to repair rectus diastasis by tightening of the abdominal muscles. Although these procedures are appealing for their shorter scars, they lack the ability to remove large amounts of excess skin, which is usually the primary issue after massive weight loss.

HERNIA REPAIR

If you need hernia repair, this repair can be performed in combination with an abdominoplasty in most cases. Hernia repair may require the surgeon to enter the abdominal cavity. Therefore, in preparation for hernia repair, you may be asked to perform a *bowel prep* with a laxative and antibiotic pills the day prior to surgery. This helps minimize the risk for bacterial contamination and infection that can occur with hernia repair.

The key to a successful hernia repair is to close the opening in the fascia with the least amount of tension; otherwise, the hernia may return. Often, to make up for a lack of adequate fascia, a synthetic mosquito net–like material called *mesh* is used for repair. After massive weight loss, however, there is usually enough loose tissue to sew the edges of the opening together. Mesh is then used to reinforce the repair as an *on-lay patch*.

Unique to umbilical hernia repair, there is a risk of having to excise the belly button if there is significant disruption of blood supply. Once fully healed from surgery, a new belly button can be created with a procedure called *neoumbilicoplasty*.

Although hernia repair is covered by insurance, this does not mean automatic approval for an abdominoplasty procedure. Usually, your plastic surgeon will be able to determine ahead of time whether you need hernia repair. However, if your skin and the underlying fat are still thick or the hernia is small, it may not be discovered until the time of surgery when there is a direct view of the entire area.

PANNICULECTOMY

A *panniculectomy* is a surgical procedure to remove only a *pannus* or *panniculus*, a large apron of skin and fat that hangs from the abdomen. A

panniculectomy is not as extensive as an abdominoplasty and can be performed more quickly than an abdominoplasty. A pannus results from obesity, but is often made worse by weight loss. The pannus is graded on a scale of one to five, according to its size.

A true panniculectomy procedure is usually reserved for individuals with a large pannus, often grade four or five. These individuals have severe disability from this hanging apron of skin and fat. For example, someone who has lost 100, maybe 200 pounds, may develop a large pannus that extends down to the mid thigh or knees. This person may still be severely obese but unable to exercise and shed any more pounds due to constant back pain from the weight of this pannus.

In some cases, a panniculectomy may be required to alleviate *panniculitis*, painful

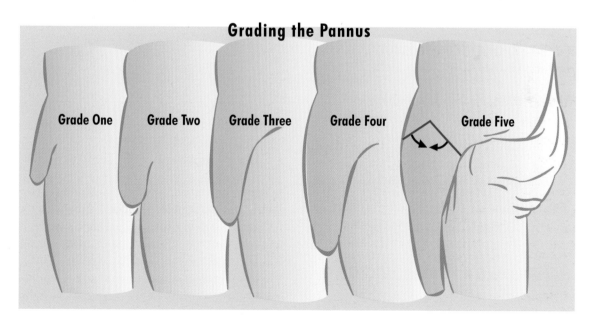

Grading the Pannus

Grade One | Grade Two | Grade Three | Grade Four | Grade Five

Grade One: Apron covers the pubic hairline. Grade Two: Apron covers the genitals in line with the upper thigh crease. Grade Three: Apron covers the upper thigh. Grade Four: Apron covers the mid thigh. Grade Five: Apron covers the knees or beyond.

Abdominoplasty

Length of Surgery:	2 to 5 hours
Type of Anesthesia:	General or deep sedation
Number of Drains:	2 to 3, usually removed within 1 to 3 weeks
Bandages:	Removed in 2 to 5 days. Abdominal binder for at least 2 weeks
Sutures:	Usually only around belly button, removed in 7 to 10 days
Swelling:	75% resolved by 6 weeks; up to 1 year for complete resolution
Duration of Hospital Stay:	1 to 2 days
Pain Level:	Moderate to severe (fascial tightening and hernia repair cause greater discomfort); prescription pain pills necessary for 10 to 14 days
Back to Work:	2 to 3 weeks, light duty
Activity Restriction:	No heavy lifting or strenuous activity for 6 weeks
Full Mature scars:	12 to 18 months
Final Result:	6 to 12 months

inflammation or infection of a pannus, prior to or at the same time as bariatric surgery in a morbidly obese individual. However, this is less commonly done because the likelihood of complications is increased when the patient is still obese.

UNDERGOING A PANNICULECTOMY

When a panniculectomy is performed, the pannus is excised. Only this large "wedge" of skin is removed. No liposuction or tightening of underlying muscles is done.

It is not uncommon for the weight of the pannus to be thirty to forty pounds.

In these cases, the stalk of the belly button is usually severely stretched and elongated, which means that its blood supply is not good; this often requires removal of the belly button along with the pannus. The risk for needing a blood transfusion is high if the pannus is very large. Just prior to suturing the incision together, drainage tubes are placed to collect fluid build-up.

The panniculectomy improves quality of life by alleviating serious functional or health problems but has limited ability to produce the best contour. Nevertheless, appearance usually does improve dramatically once the large apron of skin and fat is removed.

ABDOMINOPLASTY OR PANNICULECTOMY?

Considerable confusion surrounds the use of the terms "abdominoplasty" and "panniculectomy." You may find the terms used interchangeably, even though they are two different procedures. In large part, the confusion is due to the fact they share an identical procedural code, used for insurance reporting purposes. However, some insurance companies may be more likely to pay for a panniculectomy because abdominoplasty is usually considered a purely cosmetic procedure and carries a higher fee. In some cases, what your surgeon calls a panniculectomy may not be a true panniculectomy; you will want to clarify the terminology to determine exactly which procedure you're having.

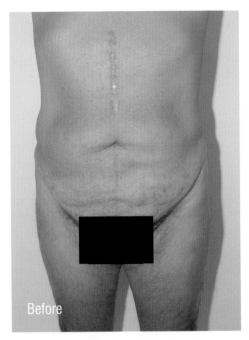

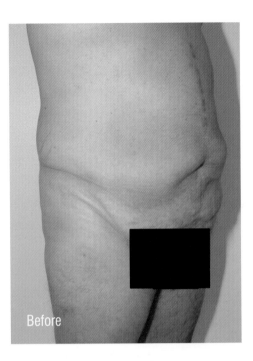

Age 53. Weight lost: 100 pounds after gastric bypass

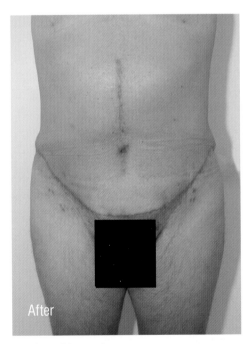

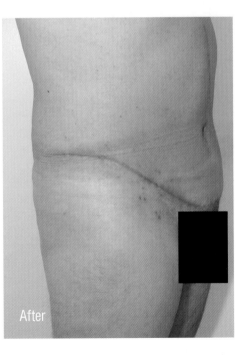

Procedure: abdominoplasty
Postoperative: 6 weeks. Preoperative BMI: 33

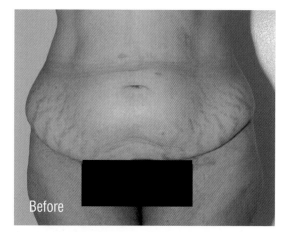

Age 57. Weight lost: 79 pounds after gastric bypass

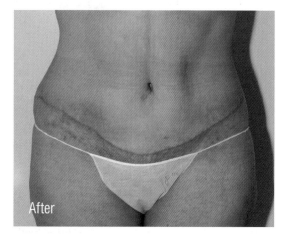

Procedure: abdominoplasty. Postoperative: 6 weeks
Preoperative BMI: 30

AFTER YOUR ABDOMINAL SURGERY

In most cases, you will spend at least one night in the hospital, surgery center, or aftercare facility for pain control. Your abdomen will be swollen and feel tight. When you stand or walk, you will need to keep your body flexed at the waist the first few days after your procedure. For the first twenty-four to forty-eight hours you are likely to require medication for moderate to severe pain. Prescription pain pills are then taken for ten to fourteen days for mild to moderate pain.

This swelling in the abdomen is normal and will last for some time. In some cases, you may even weigh a few pounds more due to water retention. It is typical for 75 percent of the swelling to have diminished by about six weeks after surgery, but it may take as long as a year to fully resolve. Any bruising will typically fade over two to three weeks.

After your surgery, it is important for you to perform deep-breathing exercises while in bed. However, your surgeon will want you up and walking as soon as possible with proper pain control and no later than the morning following surgery. As mentioned, you will have to walk slightly bent forward and should avoid any twisting motion at the waist. On occasion, muscle spasms occur if the muscles were tightened and this may require a prescription muscle relaxant. There will be temporary numbness in your abdominal region. Tingling and itching at the incision sites is normal.

RECOVERING AT HOME

Once you're home, be sure to follow your doctor's instructions for personal hygiene, wound care, and restriction of your physical activities. Your doctor will advise you to get plenty of rest but will also ask you to walk as much as you comfortably can, no less than two to three times daily. But you'll need to avoid climbing a lot of stairs the first two weeks.

Stay well hydrated, drinking a minimum of eight full glasses of water daily. Your appetite is likely to be suppressed for the first couple of weeks. Make sure you have a nutritious food plan with adequate protein intake and daily vitamin supplementation.

The final result of your surgery will take some time to be fully realized. Although you will see a vast difference immediately, there will be continued improvement over a period of months.

Wearing a Binder

You will wear an elastic abdominal binder for support and comfort for at least two weeks. On days when you are more active, you will experience more swelling at the end of the day.

Healing and Scars

It's normal for scars to be red and raised for a few weeks to months after surgery. Although they won't disappear completely, scars will fade and become less noticeable over twelve to eighteen months as they mature. It is important to avoid direct sun exposure to the scars while they are still red. This will help prevent scar darkening. Applying sunscreen with a sun protection factor (SPF) of 30 or higher will also help prevent darkening of immature scars.

Postoperative Visits

Within a week after your surgery you'll go back to the doctor's office for your first postoperative visit. Your doctor will check your incisions and may remove some drains, depending on how much fluid is still draining. On average, all of the drains are removed within one to three weeks; by this time, most fluid accumulation has stopped. It is rare for drains to remain in place for a longer period of time. Your surgeon may

have you take antibiotics while the drains are in place; these antibiotics may make you more susceptible to yeast infections.

Going Back to Work

Remember, you will not be able to drive for ten to fourteen days and as long as you are taking prescription pain pills. Expect to be back at work in two to three weeks, unless your job requires heavy lifting or vigorous physical activity, in which case you'll be advised to return to work after six weeks. Avoid any heavy lifting or strenuous activity, including sex, for at least six weeks. In general, heavy lifting means anything greater than ten pounds; this includes infants and pets. Call your doctor if you have any questions regarding your postoperative instructions or if you notice possible signs of complications.

SPECIAL CONSIDERATIONS

Pregnancy

Abdominal contouring surgery will not affect your ability to become pregnant or cause problems during pregnancy. Your skin and abdominal wall will accommodate the increase in size. However, the results from surgery may be irreversibly affected by the stretching forces of pregnancy. In most cases, however, skin excess or looseness will not return to the same degree, though you may develop abdominal bulging again. Although repeat surgery can correct this problem, you may want to wait until you are finished with childbearing before pursuing abdominal contouring surgery.

Weight Fluctuation

Weight gain or loss of more than 20 percent of your current weight may permanently affect your result. Additional weight gain is likely to go to other areas in your body; however, significant weight loss may result in sagging abdominal skin.

Breast Cancer

Be aware that a tummy tuck will eliminate the possibility of a type of breast reconstruction (after mastectomy) that uses abdominal skin and tissue to create a breast mound. Discuss this matter with your surgeon if you are at high risk for developing breast cancer and think you may require breast reconstruction at some point in the future.

RISKS OF ABDOMINOPLASTY

In addition to the risks common to all body contouring surgeries discussed earlier, the following is a list of potential complications that deserve special emphasis regarding abdominal contouring surgery.

Seroma: Despite the use of drains, this is one of the most common problems after an abdominoplasty procedure. A seroma may require additional draining; it could require surgery. If you develop a seroma, wear your abdominal binder around the clock and avoid strenuous activity for a couple of weeks after fluid withdrawal; this will minimize the chances for recurrence.

Skin Necrosis (Death of Skin): When this occurs after abdominal procedures, it most commonly occurs above the pubic area due to limited blood supply to this area. The belly button can also be affected and the risk for losing the belly button is higher following massive weight loss. Necrosis can result in delayed wound

healing, infection, additional surgery, or undesirable scarring. Your risk is highest if you are a smoker, have poorly controlled diabetes, or are significantly obese.

Recurrent Laxity: For abdominal contouring procedures done following massive weight loss, there is a greater chance of developing recurrent skin looseness or sagging that requires revisional surgery.

Issues with Fascial Tightening: Although an uncommon occurrence, the fascial tightening may come undone, with a return of abdominal bulging. This can be minimized by carefully abiding by activity restrictions. Rarely, the fascial tightening is too tight and has to be loosened surgically

---

Questions to Ask Your Surgeon

- What are my abdominal contouring options?
- Do I have a medical necessity that may qualify for insurance coverage?
- What results should I expect from the procedure?
- Do you perform hernia repair?
- What effect will surgery have on my belly button?
- What activities should I avoid for the first several weeks?
- What signs of complications should I look for?
- Under what circumstances should I call your office?

due to problems such as breathing difficulty.

Issues with Hernia Repair. Risks following repair include hernia recurrence and infection of the mesh, which requires its removal.

Deep Vein Thrombosis/Pulmonary Embolism: Potentially life-threatening, this risk is a concern following abdominoplasty. Risk can be significantly reduced by early and regular walking. In high-risk cases, injectable blood thinners are used. The risk is highest during the first couple of weeks after surgery and decreases as your activity level returns to normal.

TIPS FOR RECOVERY

- Have a second abdominal binder available. Do not wash postoperative garments in hot water or place in the dryer because they will shrink.

- Place comfortable pillows under your knees and upper back while sleeping; hug a pillow while coughing or sneezing.

- Use a heating pad or hot water bottle to help with a sore back; do not apply heat to any surgical sites unless instructed by your surgeon.

CHAPTER
8

Thigh and Buttock Contouring

Perhaps you have already had a tummy tuck and are now wondering what can be done to improve the appearance of your thighs and buttocks. With a flatter stomach and better-defined waistline, the skin excess and sagging in these areas may seem even more pronounced and out of proportion with the rest of your body. You may still be limited in the types of clothes you can fit into, or you may be bothered by the constant friction of skin rubbing between your thighs when you walk.

Under normal circumstances, the thighs and buttocks sag over time. Of course, this sagging is greatly exaggerated after massive weight loss. There may be loss of volume in the buttocks or reduced size that produce "deflation" and a less appealing silhouette. In many cases of excess weight loss, the buttocks may even be partially hidden by a large overhanging fold of skin.

Women, who are typically more pear-shaped, may show greater changes in these areas; they are also prone to cellulite formation.

THIGH LIFT

Also called a *thighplasty*, thigh lift surgery includes procedures that excise and tighten skin along both the inner and outer thighs. In most cases, these procedures are completed in two or more stages. When performing an outer thigh lift, the surgeon is able to remove the large bulge of sagging skin on the outer thigh, referred to as a *saddlebag deformity*, commonly found in women. This procedure is typically combined with a buttock lift. An inner thigh lift is then performed at a second stage.

Inner thigh lift surgery, in particular, is challenging for a number of reasons. The skin and underlying tissues of the inner thigh are thin and looser than the tissue of most other areas on your body. This weaker tissue quality makes it difficult to obtain good and long-lasting results when excess skin is removed. With contouring of the inner thigh, the incision may be long and visible, depending on the degree of excess skin and laxity along the inner thigh.

The inner thighs are significantly affected by adjoining body areas. In most cases, procedures of the central body, such as a tummy tuck or a body lift, will provide improvement to the thigh area. To obtain optimal results, it is best to stage procedures, with an inner thigh lift usually

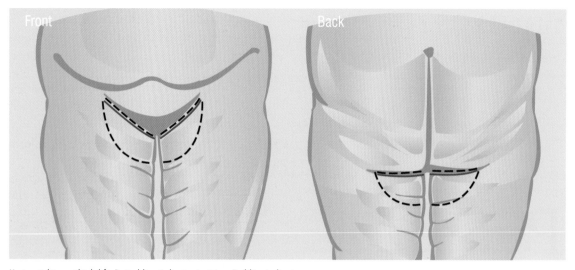

Horizontal inner thigh lift. Dotted line indicates incision. Red line indicates scar.

performed after procedures that lift the central body area. Staging is particularly important for patients with higher BMIs so that recurrent loose skin can be addressed with follow-up procedures.

There are variations of thigh lift surgery; the one your surgeon uses will depend on the nature of the excess skin on your thighs.

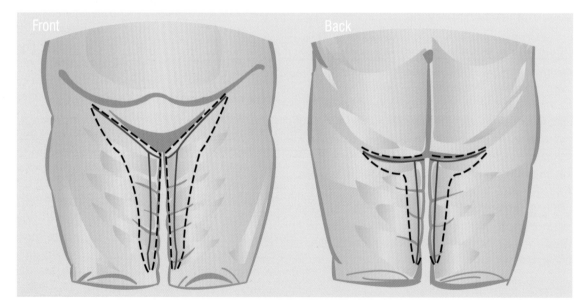

Vertical inner thigh lift

UNDERGOING AN INNER THIGH LIFT

In most cases, general anesthesia will be used for inner, or medial, thighplasty. Your surgeon may first perform liposuction to remove excess fat. Depending on the degree of skin excess, the surgeon will make an incision that runs along the groin crease; the incision may extend along the upper inner thigh and back towards the lower most fold of the buttock. With severe skin excess, an incision will also be made down the length of the inner thigh.

It is important that sutures are placed in the deep connective tissue layer for support, limiting downword migration of the scar; this prevents traction on the vagina which can lead to significant distortion. One to two surgical drains may be placed in each thigh. The wounds are covered with a light gauze dressing or sealed with tissue glue. Inner thigh lift surgery will take between two to four hours to complete.

BUTTOCK CONTOURING

In most cases, a buttock lift is performed in combination with an outer thigh lift. This contouring procedure improves the shape of your buttocks as well as skin tone.

There are also procedures available to restore projection to "deflated" buttocks. During a buttock lift, an island of tissue underlying the skin can be preserved and rearranged to provide greater fullness and a more natural shape. This is called *buttock autoaugmentation.*

There are other options to enhance the contour of the buttocks; these include insertion of solid silicone implants or taking fat from elsewhere in your body and injecting it into your buttocks. Either of these procedures may be options once you are fully healed from a buttock lift procedure. However, these procedures carry their own risks and are not widely practiced by all plastic surgeons.

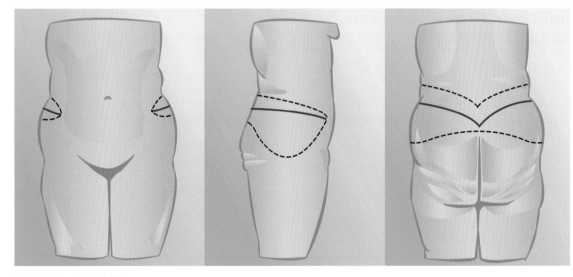

Outer thigh and buttock lift

Thigh and Buttock Lift Surgery	
Length of Surgery:	2 to 4 hours
Type of Anesthesia:	General
Number of Drains:	2 to 4, usually removed within 1 to 3 weeks
Bandages:	Removed in 2 to 5 days
Sutures:	Usually none to be removed
Swelling:	75% resolved by 6 weeks; up to 1 year for complete resolution Slower resolution for the inner thighs
Duration of Hospital Stay:	1 to 2 days
Pain Level:	Moderate to severe initially; inner thighs most painful; prescription pain pills necessary for 2 weeks
Back to Work:	2 to 4 weeks, light duty
Activity Restriction:	No heavy lifting or strenuous activity for 4 to 6 weeks
Fully Mature Scars:	12 to 18 months
Final Result:	6 to 12 months

UNDERGOING AN OUTER THIGH AND BUTTOCK LIFT

This procedure is performed under general anesthesia in most cases. The surgeon will make an incision near the top of the hip bone along the waistline to the buttock crease in the back. Liposuction is used to remove fat deposits, but more importantly, it loosens skin attachments along the outer thigh, allowing for greater lift.

If buttock autoaugmentation is performed, an island of tissue is preserved below the skin on each side; this is shaped and secured with sutures.

With weight loss, you may have developed thinning of tissues overlying your tailbone, making it uncomfortable for you to sit on hard surfaces. While performing a buttock lift, the surgeon can draw tissue over the tailbone area to provide greater padding.

At the end of the surgery, one or two surgical drains are usually placed on both sides. Light gauze dressing is used to cover the wounds. The outer thigh lift and buttock lift procedure will take four to six hours to complete.

MONSPLASTY (PUBIC LIFT)

Often after massive weight loss, severely sagging and bulky skin will be present in the pubic area, the *mons pubis*. This excess skin can be very bothersome and may even limit intimacy. A tummy tuck procedure alone may not correct this problem. If you're having an inner thigh lift, the surgeon can often remove excess skin in the pubic area; this is combined with liposuction to produce a flatter contour. This procedure is called a *monsplasty*.

INSURANCE CONSIDERATIONS

It is unlikely that insurance will cover most procedures related to the thigh and buttock areas. The decision for any coverage will be based on medical necessity. Most often, insurance will cover problems relating to excess skin along the inner thigh areas. As mentioned earlier, it is important to obtain medical documentation to present to insurance companies.

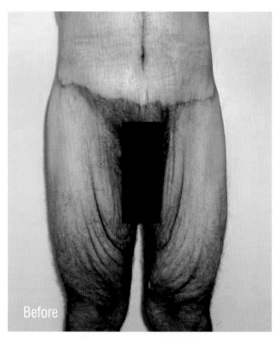

Before

Age: 40. Weight lost: 165 pounds after gastric bypass

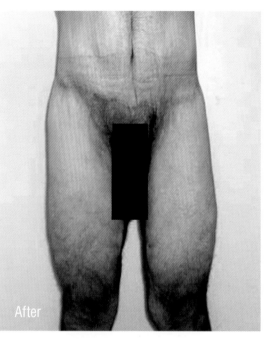

After

Procedure: Vertical inner thigh lift. Postoperative: 3 months
Patient also had a body lift. Preoperative BMI: 32

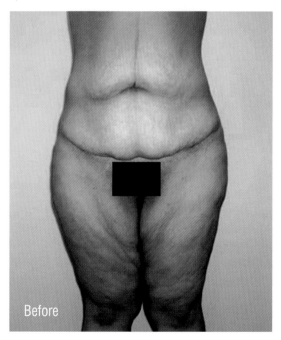

Before

Age: 33. Weight lost: 172 pounds after gastric bypass

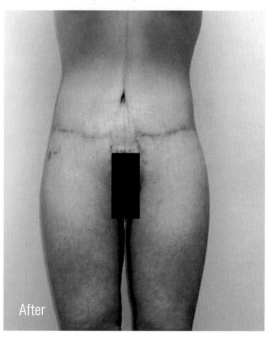

After

Procedure: Vertical inner thigh lift. Postoperative: 5 months
Patient had body lift prior to thigh lift. Preoperative BMI: 31

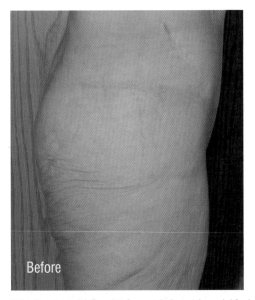

Before

Buttocks appear "deflated" after weight loss. A buttock lift alone would further flatten the buttocks.

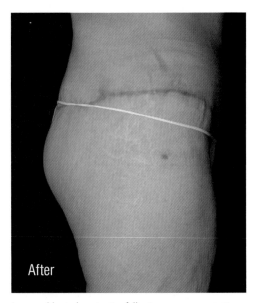

After

Increased buttock projection following autoaugmentation

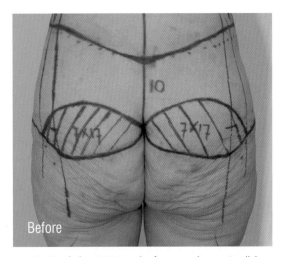

Before

Age: 50. Weight lost: 140 pounds after gastric bypass. Parallel markings indicate where tissue will be left to increase projection.

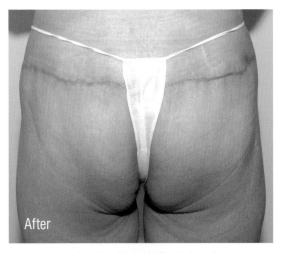

After

Procedure: Lateral thigh and buttock lift with buttock autoaugmentation
Postoperative: 2 months. Preopertive BMI: 21

AFTER YOUR SURGERY

You can expect to be in the hospital for one or two days. You may have a urinary catheter in place, especially following an inner thigh lift; this will be more convenient and comfortable for you during the first twelve to twenty-four hours. To minimize the chance for blood clot formation, you should get out of bed and begin walking as soon as possible, according to your surgeon's instructions. If you have had buttock autoaugmentation, you should lie primarily on your stomach while in bed; there may also be restrictions on sitting to avoid pressure, which can delay healing.

RECOVERING AT HOME

Do not sit or bend at the hips or knees for longer than thirty minutes at a time during the first two weeks after surgery. You will return to your doctor's office two to five days after surgery to have the dressings removed and the incisions checked. Drains are usually removed after one week. In most cases, you will be provided with a special post-operative garment or instructed to wear spandex exercise gear to provide support while the incisions heal.

Compared to other areas on the body, swelling in the inner thighs takes longer to resolve; in some cases significant swelling can persist for up to six months. If you see any signs of infection or if you are experiencing other possible complications, such as fluid buildup under your skin, call your doctor right away.

You will be able to return to work two to four weeks following surgery. Strenuous activity can usually be resumed at four to six weeks.

RISKS OF THIGH/BUTTOCK SURGERY

Tissue Edema: Tissue swelling, called lymphedema, in the legs may persist or become chronic.

Scar Migration: Scars along the inner thigh can migrate downwards away from the groin crease and become more noticeable.

Wound Separation: Small areas of the wound may open up, in particular overlying the tailbone and at the intersection of incisions.

Infection: Due to proximity to the groin area, wound infection from contamination is a greater risk.

Seroma: This is more likely to occur in the thigh area.

Recurrent Laxity: Due to the weaker tissue quality along the inner thigh, recurrent skin looseness occurs with greater frequency.

Fat Necrosis (death of fat tissue): This occurs when areas of fat underlying the skin die as a result of diminished blood supply. This is a greater risk following autoaugmentation, and may lead to firmness, surface irregularity or surgical removal.

Questions to Ask Your Surgeon

- What are my options for inner thigh lift surgery?
- Where will the scars be located?
- Am I a candidate for a combination thigh-buttock lift?
- What are options for restoring volume to my buttocks?
- Should these procedures be staged to obtain the best result?
- What are the risks of surgery?
- Will I be given general anesthesia?
- When can I go back to work?

77

The Body Lift

If you have extensive skin looseness or laxity after massive weight loss, you may feel as if you are wearing an oversized skin suit. And even though any one body contouring procedure can produce a dramatic result, one procedure alone is often not enough to create balance in your body contour. For example, flattening and tightening the abdomen with an abdominoplasty procedure does not entirely address the waistline and may actually make the hips look wider. Similarly, an abdominoplasty may also make the excess skin on the thighs stand out more.

A body lift is a newer procedure, in which the plastic surgeon uses a three-dimensional approach to blend several contouring procedures into one operation. When it is performed following massive weight loss, the result is an all-around balanced body shape. Body lift surgery can also restore body contour that has been lost due to the natural aging process, pregnancy and in situations where previous liposuction has left significant skin looseness.

WHAT IS A BODY LIFT?

A *body lift* restores contour to the midsection of the body. Most body lift procedures combine an abdominoplasty with a lift in the outer thigh and buttocks. These areas usually develop the greatest degree of deformity following massive weight loss and are often best treated simultaneously. A body lift typically results in full restoration of waistline contour, better definition of the abdomen, and tighter skin in the thighs and buttocks, often with dramatic improvement in the appearance of cellulite.

You may discover that the terms used for body lift procedures are not the same among all plastic surgeons. Other names that you may find used to describe the body lift are *lower body lift, belt lipectomy, central body lift,* and *circumferential torsoplasty.* Although there may be differences in surgeon preference, in many instances, there is significant overlap of technique. Because there is much variation in deformity, the body lift procedure and scar location may vary from individual to individual. Ultimately, the final result will provide a balanced and aesthetic look.

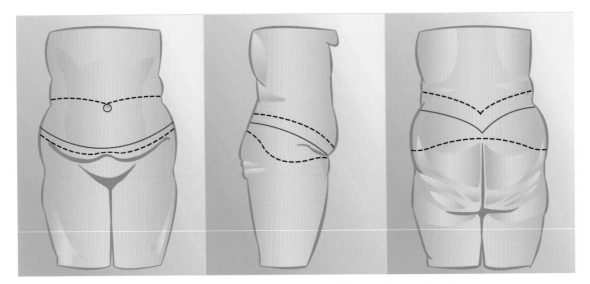

Incision placement for a body lift, which usually includes a tummy tuck, outer thigh lift, and buttock lift. Dotted line indicates incision. Red line indicates scar.

UNDERGOING A BODY LIFT

The order in which the procedures are carried out will depend on your surgeon's preference. In many cases, the abdominoplasty procedure is performed first, while you are lying flat on the operating table. Upon completion, you are then turned onto your side and the abdominoplasty incision is continued as the thigh and buttock lift incision. This process is then repeated on the opposite side. Liposuction is commonly used to remove fat deposits in the thighs, flanks, and occasionally the abdominal area. You can expect to have four to six drains placed.

At the conclusion of surgery, the incisions are typically covered with light gauze dressings. Tight dressings or elastic garments are usually avoided because they may be too constricting as normal postoperative swelling increases over the next two to three days. Significant constriction can reduce blood supply that is necessary for healing.

The length of time required for body lift surgery varies. Your procedure may last anywhere from four to eight hours.

AFTER YOUR SURGERY

Following body lift surgery, you can expect to stay two to four days in the hospital, where the staff will tend to your needs and carefully monitor your progress. The primary reason for the hospital stay is to ensure that you have proper pain control and can move around comfortably. Your waistline will be significantly swollen right after surgery; this will start to subside after approximately seventy-two hours. You will also feel tightness around your waist; be especially cautious when initially getting out of bed.

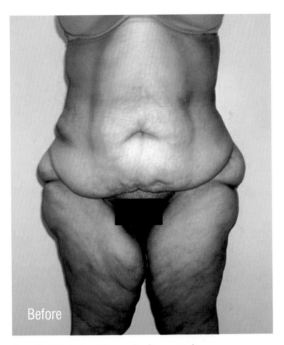

Age: 41. Weight lost: 79 pounds after gastric bypass

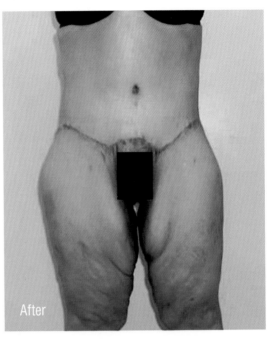

Procedure: body lift. Postoperative: 7 months
Patient is planning a thigh lift. Preoperative BMI: 31

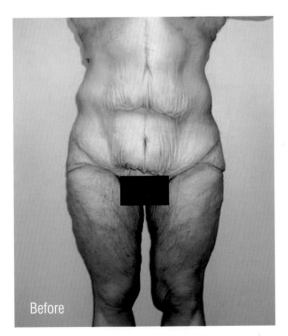

Age: 46. Weight lost: 225 pounds after gastric bypass

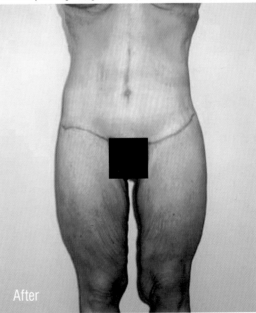

Procedure: body lift. Postoperative: 7 months
Preoperative BMI: 28

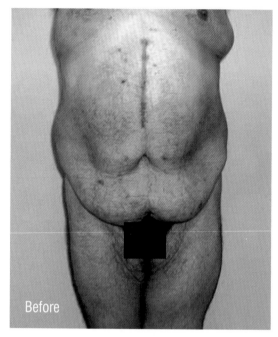

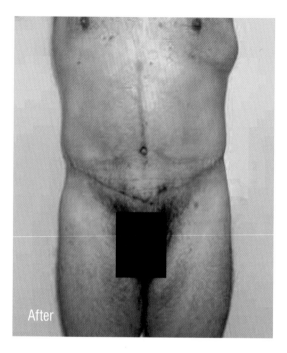

Age: 55. Weight lost: 152 pounds after gastric bypass

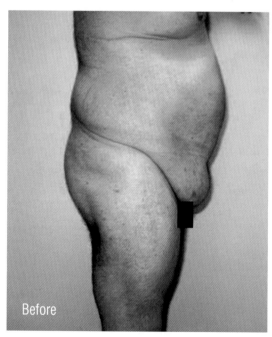

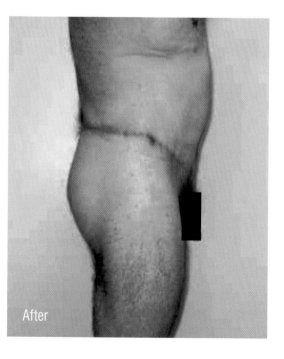

Procedure: body lift. Postoperative: 7 months
Preoperative BMI: 35

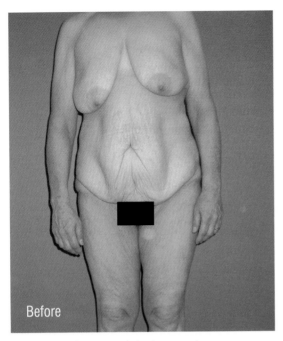

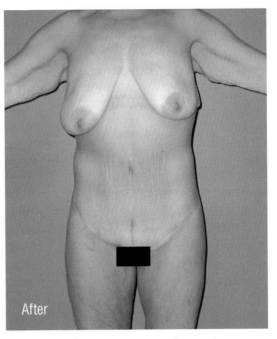

Age 45. Weight lost: 125 pounds after gastric bypass

Procedure body lift Postoperative: 10 months
Preoperative BMI: 28

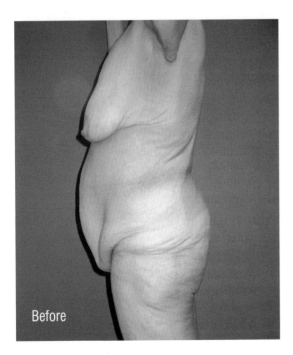

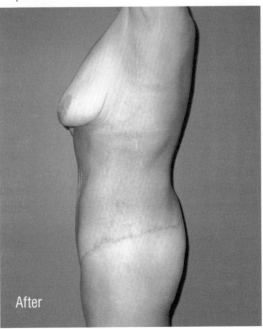

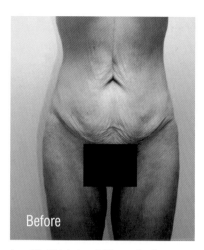
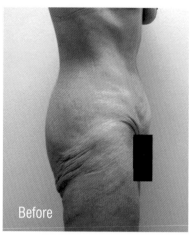
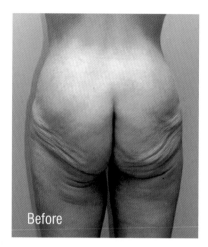

Age: 35. Weight lost: 141 pounds after gastric bypass

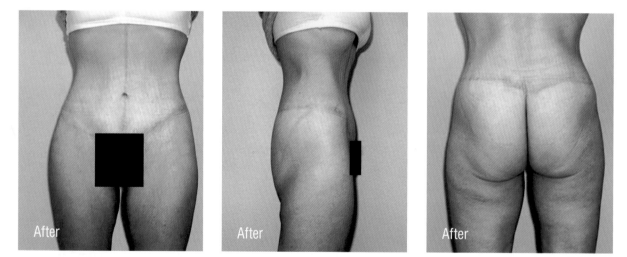

Procedure: body lift. Postoperative: 18 months
Preoperative BMI: 20

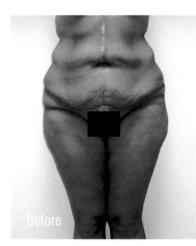
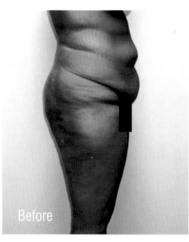
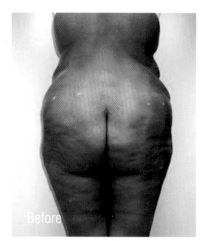

Age: 46. Weight lost: 139 pounds after gastric bypass

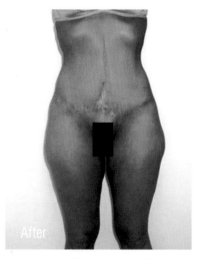
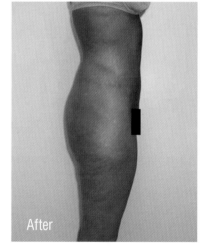
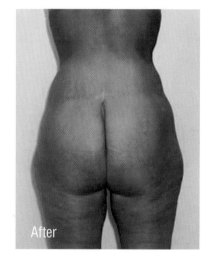

Procedure: body lift. Postoperative: 30 months
Preoperative BMI: 28. Scar near navel resulted
from skin death; patient reported a history of
smoking

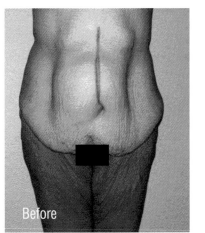 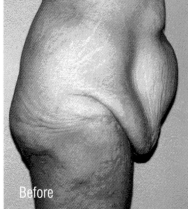 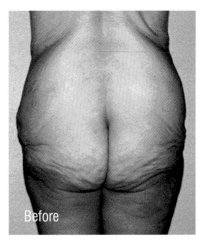

Age: 46. Weight lost: 139 pounds after gastric bypass

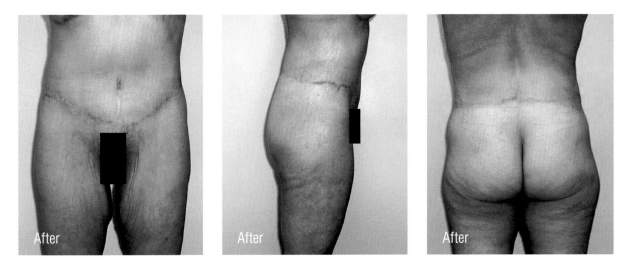

Procedure: body lift. Postoperative: 4 years
Preoperative BMI: 29

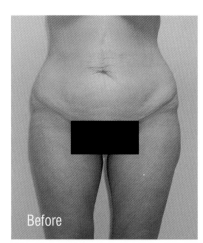
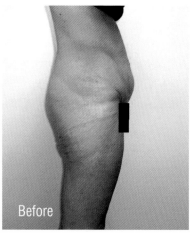
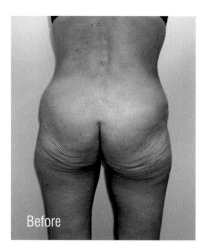

Age: 24. Weight lost: 115 pounds after gastric bypass

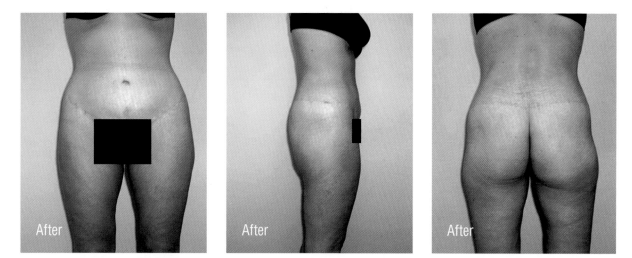

Procedure: body lift. Postoperative: 2 years
Preoperative BMI: 21

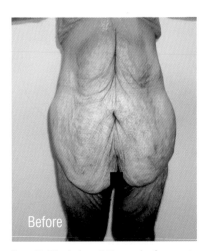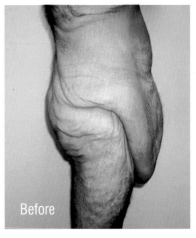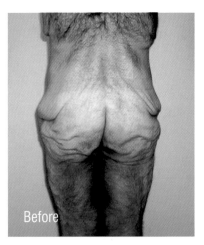

Age: 40. Weight lost: 165 pounds after gastric bypass

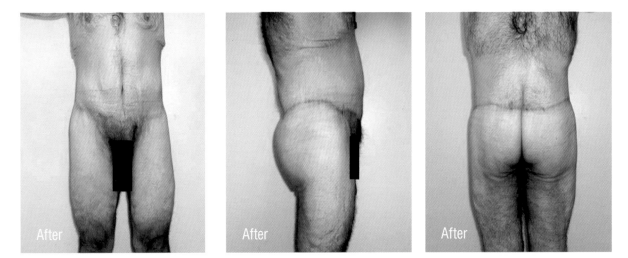

Procedure: body lift followed by inner thigh lift
Postoperative: 10 months
Preoperative BMI: 32

RECOVERING AT HOME

Naturally, your recovery period after a body lift will take longer than if you had had a tummy tuck. Initially, expect some numbness and tightness in areas that were contoured. For the first two weeks, avoid climbing up or down stairs unless it's absolutely necessary to do so.

You'll need to see your doctor one week after your procedure to have some of the drains removed; the rest are usually taken out two to three weeks after surgery. Most of your sutures will dissolve, but a few will require removal at your doctor's office, typically two weeks after your procedure.

It'll probably be at least four weeks before you can return to work. If your job involves heavy physical activity, your surgeon will ask you to wait at least six weeks before going back to work. Save any rigorous physical workouts for after your recovery period, typically eight weeks or more after your procedure.

If you're like most patients, you'll become more and more pleased with your body lift results as the weeks pass. For example, the swelling around your abdomen, thighs, and buttocks will be greatly improved by the third month after your surgery. With regular exercise and a healthful diet on your part, these results should last you for many years to come.

INSURANCE CONSIDERATIONS

It is unlikely that an insurance company will cover the full cost of a body lift. The decision for any coverage will be based on medical necessity. Most often, this will be for problems relating to an abdominal pannus. It is important to obtain medical documentation for any problems, medical or functional, that have developed with your weight loss.

STAGING VS. ONE SURGERY

A body lift procedure is an extensive operation, requiring significant recovery time. In some cases it may be best to stage the procedures over time. For example, you may decide to have an abdominoplasty procedure first, followed by a lateral thigh and buttock lift later. Although this will require more than one operation, the recovery after each procedure is quicker and less stressful on your body.

Staging the procedures may also be a better option if you have significant medical conditions, borderline malnutrition, or are age fifty-five or older. Even if you are quite healthy, the goal of reshaping your body may be best accomplished in two or three well planned stages.

TIPS FOR RECOVERY

- Consider renting an electric reclining chair (vinyl or leather).
- Use large, soft body pillows to help provide support and comfort while you are in bed.
- Allow plenty of time for your recovery, and don't push yourself during this time.

RISKS OF BODY LIFT PROCEDURES

Wound Separation: This is one of the more frequent complications. Small areas of the wound may open up. This is usually treated by packing the wound

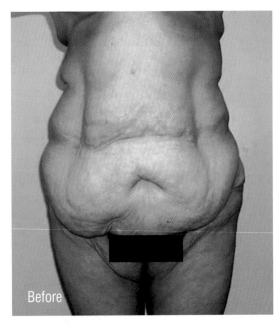

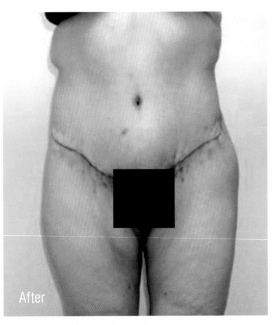

Age: 42. Weight lost: 115 pounds after lifestyle changes

Procedure: body lift. Postoperative: 4 months
Preoperative BMI: 36

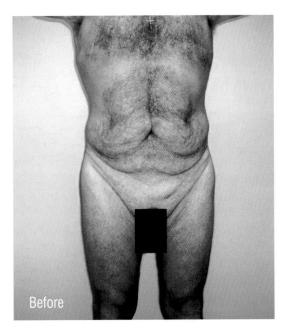

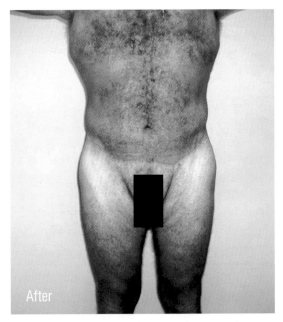

Age: 50. Weight lost: 150 pounds after gastric bypass

Procedure: body lift. Postoperative: 12 months
Preoperative BMI: 29

with gauze dressings and allowing it to heal in over two to three weeks.

Scar Complications: Incisions for body lift surgery are the most extensive. Scars may become more noticeable due to widening or asymmetry. They may also cause problems if they form a *scar contracture,* which can limit movement; or scars may itch or become painful due to hypertrophy or keloid formation. These conditions may require surgical revision.

Seroma: This may develop more frequently in the thigh area. The abdominal area is also susceptible.

Skin Necrosis (Death of Skin): The mid-portion of the back incision is under the most tension and prone to wound problems. Necrosis can result in delayed wound healing, infection, additional surgery, or unacceptable scarring.

Inadequate Lifting: Often, deformities are extreme and there is a risk of receiving an inadequate lift or having significant asymmetry requiring a second body lift for correction.

Body Lift Surgery

Length of Surgery:	4 to 8 hours
Type of Anesthesia:	General
Number of Drains:	4 to 6, usually removed within 1 to 3 weeks
Bandages:	Removed in 2 to 5 days
Sutures:	Usually only around belly button, removed in 7 to 10 days
Swelling:	75% resolved by 6 weeks; up to 1 year for complete resolution
Duration of Hospital Stay:	2 to 4 days
Pain Level:	Moderate to severe initially; prescription pain pills necessary for 2 weeks.
Back to Work:	4 to 6 weeks, light duty
Activity Restriction:	No heavy lifting or strenuous activity for 8 weeks
Fully Mature Scars:	12 to 18 months
Final Result:	6 to 12 months

Questions to Ask Your Surgeon

- What experience do you have performing body lifts?
- Which areas of my body will be affected by a body lift?
- Will I need a blood transfusion?
- Where will the scars be located?
- How many nights will I need to stay at the hospital after surgery?
- How long will the recovery period last?
- Will I need additional procedures after a body lift?

Deep Vein Thrombosis/Pulmonary Embolism: These potentially life-threatening conditions are of particular concern following body lift surgery, which is the most extensive surgery and has the longest recovery. The risk can be reduced by early and regular walking, carefully following your surgeon's guidelines. In high-risk cases, injectable blood thinners are used for prevention. The risk is highest during the first couple of weeks and decreases as your activity level returns to normal.

CHAPTER 10

Restoring Shape to Female Breasts

If you're a woman, you realize that breasts naturally begin to sag as part of the normal aging process. But regardless of your age, if you've had major weight loss, your breasts may appear "deflated." Of the skin laxity problems that occur as a result of dramatic weight loss, many women find sagging breasts to be the most troublesome.

Fortunately, there are effective procedures available to plastic surgeons to restore a more natural and rejuvenated breast. The basic types of breast surgery for which a woman may be a candidate are: breast lift, breast lift with augmentation, or breast reduction, if breasts are too large.

BREAST LIFT

A breast lift, also known as a *mastopexy*, involves lifting and reshaping the breast primarily by removing excess skin. The skin surrounding breast tissue functions like a bra that provides support. When the skin stretches and loses its elastic properties, this "bra" is no longer able to provide the necessary support to maintain the shape and position of the breast. This loss of elasticity is often evident by severe stretch marks along the upper part of the breast, which reflects damage to the skin.

How much should the breasts be lifted? It depends on the extent of *ptosis* (pronounced: toe-sis), the medical term for drooping or sagging. The degree of ptosis is classified by the relationship between the nipple and the inframammary fold, the crease where the underside of the breast meets the rib cage. With a youthful breast, the nipple and most of the breast tissue lie above this fold.

Degrees of Ptosis

- First degree (mild ptosis): The nipple lies at the level of the fold.

- Second degree (moderate ptosis): The nipple is below the fold but is still above the lowest part of the breast.

- Third degree (severe ptosis): The nipple lies below the fold and at the lower part of the breast.

- Pseudoptosis: The nipple is above the inframammary fold; however most of the breast tissue lies below it.

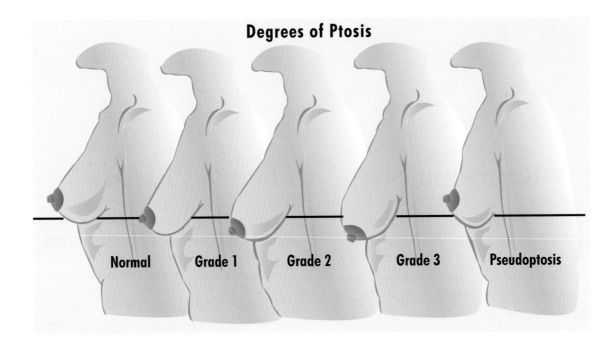

Degrees of Ptosis

Normal   Grade 1   Grade 2   Grade 3   Pseudoptosis

UNDERGOING A BREAST LIFT

The greater the droop of the breast, the greater the amount of skin that needs to be removed in order to elevate the nipple. Consequently, the removal of more skin means the surgeon will need to make extensive incisions, resulting in more scarring. In many cases, removal of excess skin alone does not permit the surgeon to form an attractive breast mound; your surgeon may also need to remove a small amount of tissue to form a shapely breast. With the removal of a significant amount of skin, the breasts could be as much as one cup size smaller.

To perform a breast lift, your surgeon will use one of several types of incisions. The type of incision used depends upon the size of the breasts and the severity of the droop. Often, the diameter of the areola is made smaller to be more proportional to the breast.

If you're a candidate for a breast lift, you may wish to talk to your surgeon about combining your breast lift with a procedure called an upper body lift, as discussed in chapter 11.

Anchor Technique

The *anchor technique* gets its name from the anchor-shaped scar it leaves on the breasts. This anchor incision is the most commonly used following massive weight loss, when the degree of ptosis is severe and requires extreme skin removal. This procedure has the ability to correct the greatest degree of sag by using both vertical and horizontal skin excisions below the nipple. The horizontal incision can be continued along the side to remove excess tissue that extends either towards the back or the underarm.

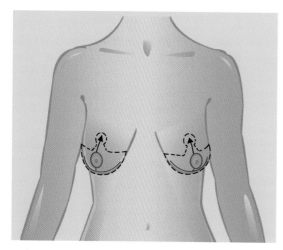

Anchor incision. Dotted line indicates incision. Red line indicates scar.

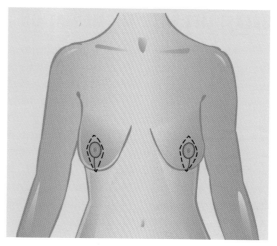

Vertical "lollipop" incision

Vertical Mastopexy

For a *vertical mastopexy*, the surgeon uses what is sometimes referred to as the "lollipop technique," because the incision and resulting scar is shaped like a lollipop. The incision circles the *areola* and then travels under the nipple and areola vertically. This approach works better for women with mild to moderate droop in which the nipple is near the inframammary fold.

Limited Breast Lift Procedures

If your breast size is small or you have less sagging, you may be a candidate for either a *crescent mastopexy* or a *doughnut mastopexy*. These procedures involve a semi-circular or circular incision around the areola only. The ability to remove excess skin is limited and these procedures are useful only for treating milder degrees of ptosis.

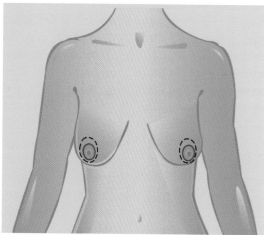

Doughnut (circumareolar) incision

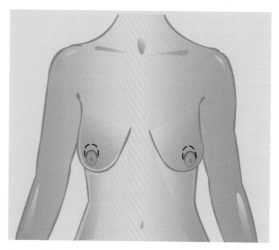

Crescent incision

BREAST LIFT WITH AUGMENTATION

About half the women who undergo a breast lift after weight loss do well with a breast lift alone. However, others will need breast augmentation—implants—along with their lift. Why is this so? Some women do not have enough breast tissue to form a normal-looking breast, especially in the upper part of the breasts; as a result, a breast lift alone will not be sufficient. An *augmentation mastopexy* procedure will be able to lift as well as provide volume, restoring a more natural contour to the breasts.

If implants are to be inserted during your breast lift, they will be inserted through the incisions used for the breast lift. The breast can then be lifted and the skin tailored properly to conform to the implants. In some cases, the procedure is best done in two stages. Depending on your unique physical characteristics and size goals, your plastic surgeon will have clear recommendations.

Some women ask if fat from elsewhere on their body can be harvested and used to increase the size of their breasts. Although possible, the injection of fat into your breast tissue is not a recommended or an accepted practice, since it could significantly hinder or prevent the early detection of breast cancer. However, you may wish to ask your surgeon about newer mastopexy techniques, such as autologous augmentation, which use rolls of skin and fat on the side of the breast to make the breast larger.

Implant Size

How big should the implants be? This can be difficult for you to estimate since cup size is not standardized and can vary between bra styles and manufacturers. Nevertheless, it is important for you to convey to your plastic surgeon how you want your breast to look. It's a good idea to select pictures from magazines that approximate your breast size goals and then take them to your initial consultation. Based on your examination, your surgeon will also have ideas and recommendations regarding implant size that is proportional to your body.

In estimating implant size, it is often helpful to select from before and after photos of other patients. Your plastic surgeon may even have implants of various sizes available in the office that you can try in your desired bra size.

Ultimately, the decision is yours. Keep in mind, however, that larger implants require your tissue to support more weight, which may mean a greater risk for problems, such as the implant displacing downward.

Implant Types
Saline

Although the outer shell of all breast implants is made of solid silicone, the majority of implants used for breast enlargement in the United States contain saline. Saline is a sterile salt solution that the surgeon uses to fill the implant at the time of surgery. If saline later leaks from the implant it is absorbed by the body without problem.

Compared to silicone gel implants, saline implants can be implanted through smaller incisions, and also allow for adjustments in the final volume or size of the implant. There are even saline implants that are adjustable for a limited period of time after surgery, allowing for the addition or

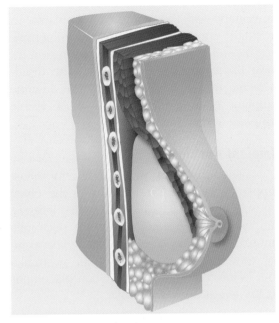

Submuscular placement of implant

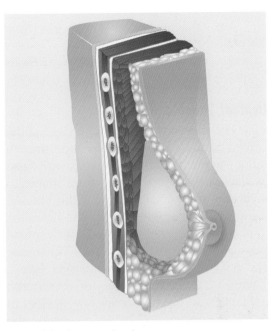

Subglandular placement of implant

removal of saline in a simple office procedure.

Saline implants in general produce excellent results. However, compared to silicone gel, they are a slightly heavier implant with a firmer feel. Often, the lower edge of the implant can be felt or produces visible wrinkling at the skin surface.

Silicone

For most people, silicone implants have a more natural look and feel. However, silicone implants have been surrounded by controversy since 1992, when concerns arose over a linkage between silicone implants and connective tissue disorders, including autoimmune diseases such as lupus and rheumatoid arthritis. As a result, the Food and Drug Administration (FDA) restricted the use of silicone gel implants. Subsequent extensive scientific studies have failed to associate silicone implants with connective tissue disorders.

Silicone gel implants are currently the most popular type of breast implant in use outside of the United States. In the United States they are FDA-approved for use only in limited clinical trials involving women who need breast reconstruction or correction of congenital breast asymmetries. You may also qualify for silicone gel implants if you have sagging breasts that require a breast lift and placement of an implant.

The newer silicone gel implants have stronger shells, as well as a more solid silicone gel consistency that makes the silicone less likely to seep into surrounding tissues. Some silicone implants also have a double shell that allows partial filling of the implants with saline.

97

The potential drawbacks to using silicone gel implants include greater expense and the need for larger incisions for placement.

Implant Shape and Texture

The most common implant used in the United States today is the round, smooth saline implant. Saline implants are also available in contoured or teardrop shapes to conform more naturally to the breast. Although appealing, contoured saline implants have not enjoyed widespread popularity, in part because they can rotate and lead to an abnormally shaped breast. There is a greater role for contoured implants with the newer silicone devices in which *cohesive gel* helps maintain the teardrop shape, allowing the surgeon greater flexibility in shaping the breast.

Both saline and silicone implants come in a variety of profiles—low, moderate, and high—which can alter projection of the breast and also allow a more accurate fit in cases where the chest is either excessively wide or narrow.

Compared to smooth implants, those that are textured have an irregular surface, preventing the implant from moving. This is important for the contoured implants. A textured implant will also be less vulnerable to *capsular contracture*, the formation of scar tissue around the implant. The disadvantage to a textured surface with a saline implant is a greater likelihood of visible rippling at the skin surface.

Implant Position

The implant position refers to breast implant placement in relation to the chest muscle, called the *pectoralis muscle*. Implants can be placed below the pectoralis muscle, in which case they are *subpectoral*, or, they may be placed above the pectoralis but below the breast tissue. Such placement is known as *subglandular*.

Most surgeons prefer subpectoral placement for several reasons. There is less chance of feeling the lower edge of the implant or seeing wrinkles at the surface since the muscle covers the implant. Additionally, in the subpectoral position, the rate of capsular contracture is lower and there is less interference of breast tissue evaluation with subsequent mammograms.

Disadvantages to placement below the muscle include a longer recovery period with more discomfort and the chance for

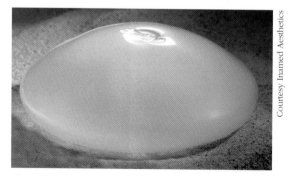

The round, smooth implants are most commonly used for breast augmentation.

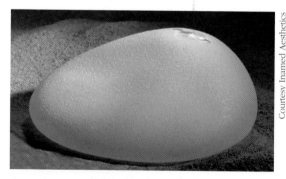

The contoured (teardrop) implant shown here has a textured surface.

Courtesy Inamed Aesthetics

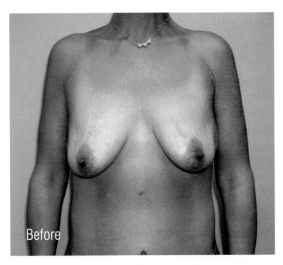

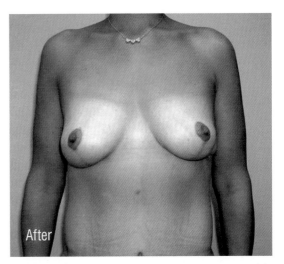

Age 40. Weight lost: 178 pounds after gastric bypass

Procedure: anchor breast lift. Postoperative: 8 months
Preoperative: BMI 31

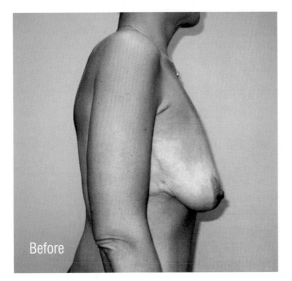

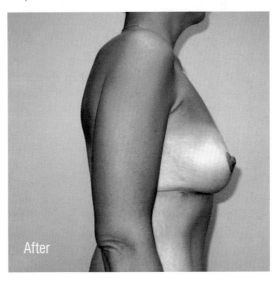

altering the shape of the implant with contraction of your chest muscles. You also can get the "double bubble" effect in which the breast continues to sag while the subpectorally placed implant remains stationary, creating a double silhouette.

To avoid this effect, a patient who has had massive weight loss may be a better candidate for subglandular placement of the implant. In this case, silicone implants should be considered as they feel more natural.

Implant-Related Risks
Capsular Contracture

This is one of the most common problems with breast implants and the most frequent reason for requiring additional

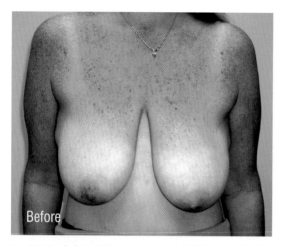

Age 37. Weight lost: 178 pounds after Lap-BAND

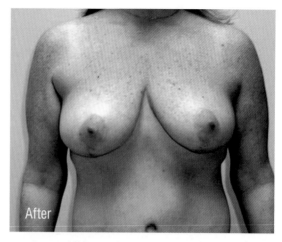

Procedure: anchor breast lift. Postoperative: 14 months
Preoperative BMI: 28

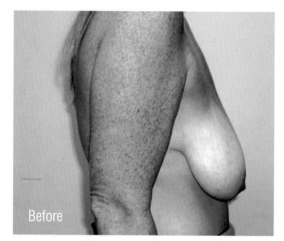

Before

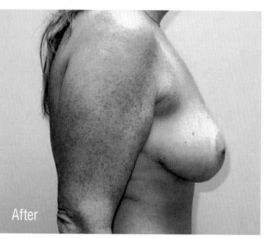

After

surgery following implant placement. As part of your body's natural response, a thin layer of scar tissue will normally form around a breast implant. Although the exact reasons are not known, this scar tissue formation can be exaggerated and result in a tight capsule that surrounds the implant. This capsule can squeeze the implant, resulting in displacement, distortion, or pain. Capsular contracture may require removal or replacement of the implant.

Deflation/Rupture

According to the FDA, a saline breast implant will have a deflation rate of 1 to 5 percent during the first three years. Manufacturers typically offer a new implant at no charge and may contribute to the replacement cost as well if failure occurs within five years.

Wrinkling

Surface irregularities, such as wrinkling, are more common with saline

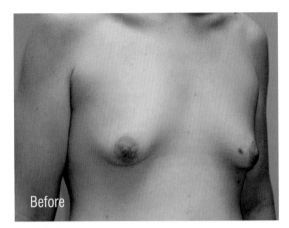

Age: 28. Weight lost: 135 pounds after gastric bypass

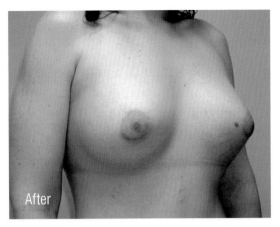

Procedure: breast augmentation with periareolar incision. Implant placement: submuscular. Postoperative: 4 months. Preoperative BMI: 26

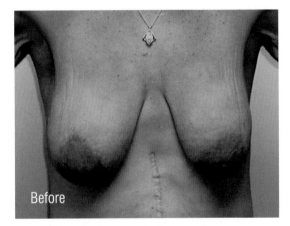

Age: 38. Weight lost: 140 pounds after gastric bypass

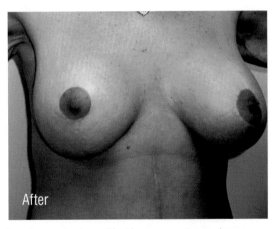

Procedure: anchor breast lift with augmentation. Implant placement: submuscular. Postoperative: 24 months Preoperative BMI: 31

implants than with silicone. This may result in patient dissatisfaction and the need for revisional surgery. In some instances, the only way to eliminate wrinkles is to remove or replace the implant.

Infection

The risk for implant infection is low. However, if infection occurs, it may require hospitalization, prolonged antibiotic

therapy, or removal of the implant. If removed, the implant cannot be replaced for a minimum of three months.

Hematoma

The risk for developing a collection of blood around the implant is also low. However if hematoma does occur around the implant, a surgical procedure may be required. Hematoma can increase the chance for developing a capsular contracture.

Implants and Breast Cancer Screening

If you are over thirty, you will probably be asked to have a mammogram prior to any breast surgery. Breast contouring procedures, including the placement of breast implants, do not increase the risk for developing breast cancer. They may, however, produce changes within the breast that need to be distinguished from cancer or pre-cancerous lesions. Most surgeons will advise against breast implants if you are at high risk for breast cancer (if you have a strong family history of it).

Following breast implant placement, a special mammogram needs to be performed with "displacement" views to properly evaluate the breast tissue. If you have breast implants, be sure to tell the radiologist who performs your mammograms.

Implant Lifespan

Note that breast implants are not expected to last for a lifetime. There is a good chance that you will require additional surgery for replacement or removal of the implants at some point. In addition, you may require additional surgery if you are unhappy with the size or shape. Talk to your surgeon about such matters.

BREAST REDUCTION

You may consider your breasts too large even after massive weight loss. Be sure that this perception is not due to severe sagging that needs correction with a breast lift. If you do suffer from medical or functional problems due to the weight of your breasts, you are likely a candidate for a breast reduction procedure, known as a *reduction mammaplasty.*

Problems with large, heavy breasts may include shoulder and neck pain, bra straps that dig into your shoulders and leave deep grooves, numbness in your hands, rash or irritation beneath your breasts, and restriction in your ability to be physically active. In addition to alleviating these problems by significantly reducing the size and weight of the breast, a breast reduction procedure will also restore breast position, shape, and perhaps symmetry.

UNDERGOING A BREAST REDUCTION

Most breast reduction procedures are performed on an outpatient basis with an overnight hospital stay. The types of incision used to perform a breast reduction are very similar to those used to perform a breast lift. And again, the incision used will depend on the size and shape of your breasts.

The anchor technique allows for removal of a large amount of breast tissue and moves the nipple and areola to a higher and more youthful position. With large breast reductions, this technique can produce a natural-looking breast shape, although the scars are the most extensive. The vertical reduction technique offers the advantage of less scarring; however, it is less useful for large breast reductions and there is usually temporary bunching of skin along the bottom portion of the scar, which occasionally requires revision.

As the surgeon performs the breast reduction, he or she will weigh any tissue removed to maintain symmetry with the opposite breast. Liposuction may be used to remove fat that extends around the sides of the breast. Any breast tissue that is removed is sent for examination by a pathologist to make sure there are no abnormal changes.

Just prior to closure, you will be placed in a seated position to check for symmetry. Any minor adjustments are then made. Depending on the procedure, you may have a small drain placed and the incisions will be closed with several layers of sutures. A light dressing is applied to the incisions, and depending on the procedure, you will be placed in an elastic wrap or a support bra.

In cases where the breasts are extremely large and long, it may be necessary to preserve the nipple and areola by removing them and placing them back into place as a graft to the newly-shaped breast mound. This is referred to as a *free nipple transfer*. In this case, however, sensation in the nipple and areola is lost and there is a greater chance for having an abnormally shaped or discolored nipple and areola. Breast-feeding following free nipple transfer is not possible.

Breast Contouring Surgery

Length of Surgery:	1 to 4 hours
Type of Anesthesia:	General or Sedation
Number of Drains:	Variable; in many cases none
Bandages:	Removed in 2 to 5 days
Sutures:	Usually only around the areola, removed in 7 to 10 days
Swelling:	75% resolved by 6 weeks; up to 1 year for complete resolution
Duration of Hospital Stay:	Either home the same day or overnight stay
Pain Level:	Mild to moderate initially; prescription pain pills necessary for up to 10 days
Back to Work:	1 to 2 weeks
Activity Restriction:	No heavy lifting or strenuous activity for 3 to 4 weeks
Fully Mature Scars:	12 to 18 months
Final Result:	6 to 12 months

INSURANCE CONSIDERATIONS

Reduction mammaplasty may qualify for insurance coverage if the operation is performed out of medical necessity. With documentation of medical problems, some companies will pay based on the amount of breast tissue removed; this usually means removal of at least 500 grams of tissue, about one pound per breast (one pound equals 454 grams). Other companies use complex formulas to compare the size of the breasts with the overall size of the body.

AFTER YOUR BREAST LIFT OR REDUCTION

On average, you can expect mild to moderate pain, which decreases significantly after a few days and is mostly gone within three to four weeks. Expect your breasts to appear swollen and feel heavy and firm after surgery. There will be gradual softening over a period of months. Bruising is usually minimal.

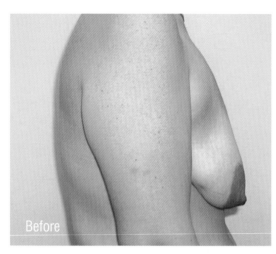

Age: 41. Weight lost: 170 pounds after gastric bypass

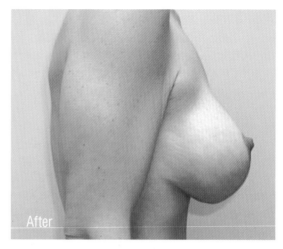

Procedure: vertical breast lift with augmentation. Implant placement: submuscular. Postoperative: 3 months. Preoperative BMI: 30

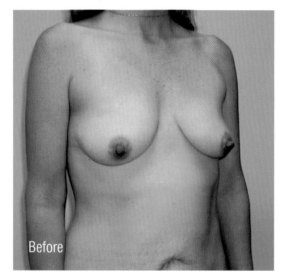

Age: 36. Weight lost: 90 pounds after gastric bypass

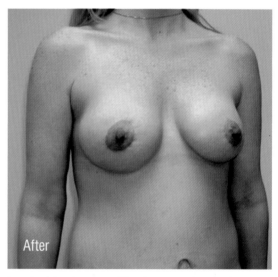

Procedure: doughnut breast lift with augmentation. Implant placement: submuscular. Postoperative: 2 months. Preoperative BMI: 26

Follow-up Care

Have a sports bra available to wear postoperatively if your surgical bra gets soiled. Underwire bras are usually discouraged.

Your surgeon will remove the dressing during your first follow-up visit, as well as any drainage tubes. You will be asked to continue wearing a support bra.

During the first few days it is best to sleep in an elevated position. Avoid sleeping on your stomach for the first two weeks after surgery. To minimize swelling and the risk for bleeding, do not bend over, strain, exercise, or do any other activities that could increase pressure in your chest during the first week. You will probably be able to drive within one week and be back at work within one to two weeks. Most strenuous activities can be resumed at three to four weeks.

As you heal, it is normal to experience burning, tingling, and shooting pains. Most breast numbness is temporary but may take months or even up to a year or more to resolve.

Pregnancy and Breast-feeding Considerations

Pregnancy will cause your breasts to enlarge and may result in recurrent sagging. Although breastfeeding is possible in most cases following breast contouring procedures, there is a chance that it could be limited. Consider delaying a breast contouring surgery if you are planning on becoming pregnant.

RISKS OF BREAST CONTOURING SURGERY

Sensory Change: In most cases, changes in skin sensation following breast surgery are temporary. However, there is a chance of permanent change, including numbness and hypersensitivity, which can be most problematic with the nipple and areola.

Asymmetry: Most individuals are not perfectly symmetric. Your plastic surgeon will likely point out any subtle differences

that exist prior to surgery. Following breast surgery, asymmetry may become more obvious. Revisional surgery may be necessary.

Tissue Necrosis (Death of Tissue): Breast procedures involve interrupting blood supply to tissues. In some cases, this may be enough to result in the death and loss of tissue, such as the nipple and areola, breast skin, or breast tissue. Necrosis can result in delayed wound healing, infection, hardening of the breast, additional surgery or unacceptable scarring. Individuals who smoke have a much higher chance for this to occur.

Abnormal Scar Formation: Scars can be quite extensive for breast procedures that provide a lot of lift or significant breast reduction. Although incisions on the breast heal favorably most of the time, there is a risk of developing noticeable scars. This may require further treatment or scar revision.

Questions to Ask Your Surgeon

- What are my surgical options for restoring breast shape?
- Where will the scars be?
- Will I need augmentation with a breast lift?
- Will the implants go above or below the muscle?
- What kind of implants do you prefer to use?
- How do you determine implant size?
- What are the risks of surgery?
- Will I be given general anesthesia?
- Will I be able to breastfeed after this procedure?

CHAPTER 11

Arm, Chest, and Upper Body Lifts

As you realize, massive weight loss often produces a "curtain" of loose skin around the entire body. It's not uncommon for this sagging skin across the chest to connect with large skin folds extending onto the upper back. Being uncomfortable with these changes is natural. For many individuals following weight loss, the skin laxity in the upper body is an area of great concern.

A number of procedures can effectively restore your upper body contour. In this chapter we'll first discuss procedures for contouring the arms and then discuss contouring the male chest area. We'll also discuss a procedure, the upper body lift, in which all these areas are contoured in one surgical procedure.

ARM LIFTS

If you have severe skin excess hanging from your upper arms, you are a likely candidate for an arm contouring procedure called a *standard brachioplasty*. During this procedure, your surgeon can remove a significant amount of excess skin and fat tissue. The scar for this procedure runs along the inner arm from the underarm to the elbow, and in certain circumstances onto the forearm. The procedure that additionally removes excess underarm skin is referred to as an *extended brachioplasty*. In this case, the scar traverses the underarm to the side of the chest. It is important to have a clear understanding and acceptance of scar location prior to proceeding with surgery.

If you have only a mild amount of skin excess at the uppermost part of the arm, your surgeon may be able to perform a *short-scar brachioplasty*. Here, the surgeon confines the scar to the upper one-third of the inner arm and axilla, the armpit area; however, this procedure is typically not adequate for the majority of individuals who have had significant weight loss.

The skin quality found along the inner arm is similar to that of the inner thigh area. With severe degrees of skin excess it may not be possible to obtain a desirable result with a single operation, and the chance for recurrent skin looseness is significant. Planning to have more than one procedure allows the surgeon greater opportunity to obtain the best possible result.

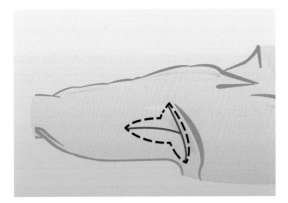

Arm lift short or "T" incision

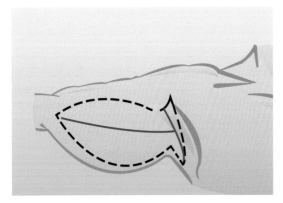

Arm lift standard incision

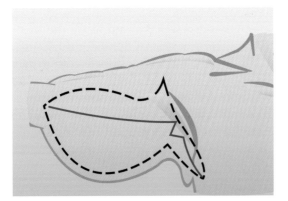

Arm lift extended incision

UNDERGOING AN ARM LIFT PROCEDURE

General anesthesia is usually preferred for extensive brachioplasty procedures. Liposuction is performed to remove fatty deposits, allowing for better reshaping of the arm and shoulder area. Skin and underlying soft tissue is then excised, using skin markings placed prior to surgery as a guide. When incisions cross a joint (such as the shoulder or elbow), a Z-shaped incision is often used to prevent the scar from contracting and limiting movement. The resulting scar is shaped like the letter "Z". As a final step, additional liposuction may be used to further contour the arm.

At the end of the procedure, a surgical drain may be placed. The wound is closed with several layers of sutures for maximum support. Most surgeons prefer to have the patient wear a compression garment to support the incision and minimize swelling. The brachioplasty procedure will take two to three hours to complete. In most cases, it is an outpatient procedure.

AFTER ARM CONTOURING SURGERY

In most cases, it's safe to use your arms right away for routine activities, such as eating; however, your doctor will most likely ask you to avoid reaching up or stretching your arms outward and upward during the first two weeks after surgery. Avoiding prolonged flexion at the elbows and keeping your arms elevated on pillows while in bed is important in reducing postoperative swelling.

You will return to your doctor's office two to five days after surgery to have the dressings removed and the incisions checked. Drains are also usually removed within two to five days. You can return to work within one to two weeks following brachioplasty and be able to resume strenuous activity within four to six weeks.

Here are some additional recommendations if you are planning to have an arm lift. During a consultation, ask your surgeon to draw the outline of expected scars on your inner arm or chest with a marking pen. This will allow you to assess the location of scars for a few days to determine if they will be acceptable to you.

After your surgery, wear the compression garment for the amount of time recommended by your surgeon to ensure the best possible contour for arms, and chest, too, if you've had a chest or breast procedure.

Remember the importance of avoiding sun exposure of your incision sites for as long as the scars are still red. Sun exposure will result in darkening with a more conspicuous scar. If you must expose these areas to sun, apply a sunscreen with a sun protection factor (SPF) of 30 or higher.

Chest Contouring for Men

If you're a man, you were likely embarrassed by the size of your breasts when you were overweight. And now, even after weight loss, you're probably self-conscious about the sagging skin on your chest. Most obese men accumulate fat along the chest and some develop breast gland enlargement, a condition called *gynecomastia*. Although obesity is a common cause, other medical conditions as well as certain drugs can produce gynecomastia. These should be evaluated and treated prior to proceeding with surgery for gynecomastia.

As weight is lost, breast deformity results from a combination of enlarged breast glandular tissue and excess fat and skin. If this is your situation, you can benefit from the excision of excess skin, fat, and glandular tissue. Although this can provide for a more masculine shape, scars on the chest may be obvious.

UNDERGOING MALE CHEST CONTOURING

Contouring of the male chest following massive weight loss is usually performed under general anesthesia. The procedure typically begins with ultrasound-assisted liposuction, which is effective at reducing the amount of fatty and glandular tissue in the male breast. Removal of this tissue will help the skin over the chest assume a more natural contour.

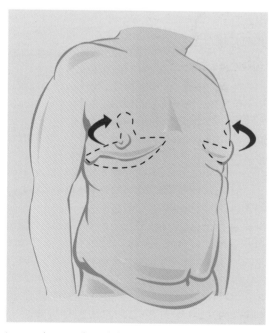

Incision placement for male breast reduction

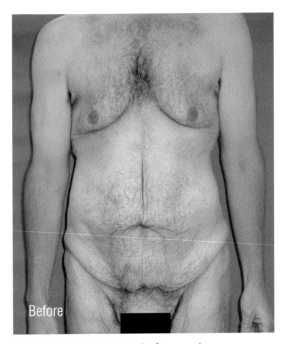

Before

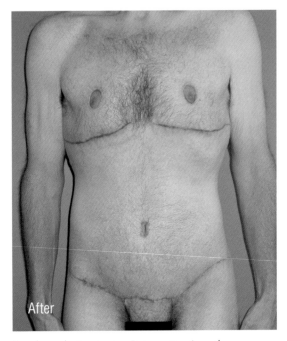

After

Age: 45. Weight lost: 200 pounds after gastric bypass

Procedures: chest contouring. Postoperative: 6 months
Patient also had a body lift. Preoperative BMI: 27

In most cases, an incision is placed along the natural crease at the base of the breasts. The same incision may extend towards the side or flank areas to address skin and fat excess in these areas. In addition, there is likely to be an incision around the nipple and in some cases a vertical scar as well, creating an inverted "T" scar. In addition, the nipple can be restored to a more natural location. In cases where there is only breast gland enlargement and no skin excess, the scar can be confined to around the nipple.

A surgical drain may be placed on each side of the chest. The incisions are closed with several layers of sutures, and a compression garment is placed for support and to minimize swelling. The procedure will take two to three hours to complete. A chest contouring procedure is typically done on an outpatient basis.

After Male Breast Reduction Surgery

Discomfort following male chest contouring surgery is usually mild. Swelling and numbness will improve significantly over four to six weeks but will take months to completely resolve. It is important to wear the compression garment as instructed, usually for two to four weeks. Light duty work can usually be resumed at one to two weeks and strenuous activity or exercise at four to six weeks.

UPPER BODY LIFT

An upper body lift is a procedure to remove excess skin and restore contour to the upper back, the sides of the chest, and the breasts—for both women and men. Some surgeons combine even more procedures into one operation, including

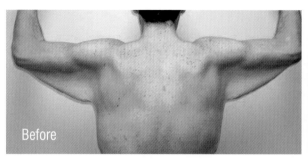

Before

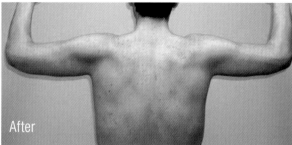

After

Age: 37. Weight lost: 270 pounds after gastric bypass

Procedure: arm lift. Postoperative: 6 months
Preoperative BMI: 33

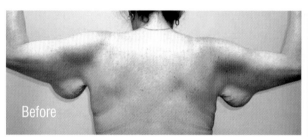

Before

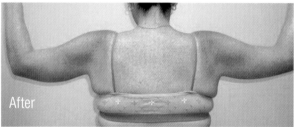

After

Age: 33. Weight lost: 110 pounds after gastric bypass

Procedure: arm lift. Postoperative: 3 months
Preoperative BMI: 31

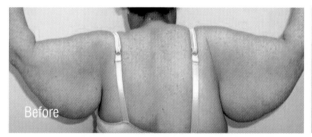

Before

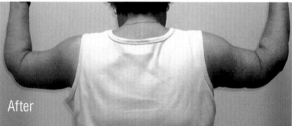

After

Age: 58. Weight lost: 80 pounds after gastric bypass

Procedure: arm lift. Postoperative: 5 months
Preoperative BMI: 37

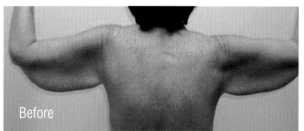

Before

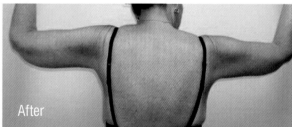

After

Age: 50. Weight lost: 140 pounds after gastric bypass

Procedure: arm lift. Postoperative: 5 months
Preoperative BMI: 25

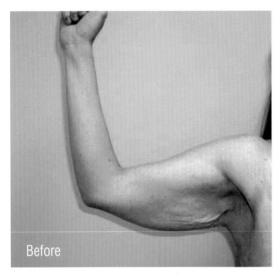

Before

Age: 30. Weight lost: 130 pounds after gastric bypass

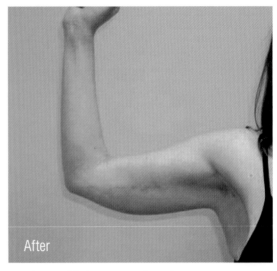

After

Procedure: armlift. Postoperative: 9 months
Preoperative BMI: 26

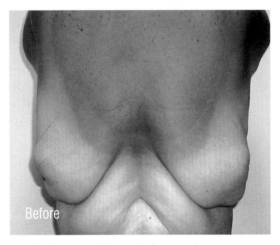

Before

Age: 30. Weight lost: 155 pounds after gastric bypass

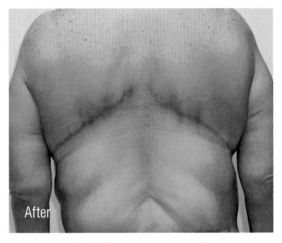

After

Procedure: upper body lift. Postoperative: 6 months
Preoperative BMI: 30

contouring of the arms. Since the current definitions of upper body lift surgery differ among plastic surgeons, make sure you fully understand what your upper body lift will address.

Upper body lifts are playing a greater role in contouring the individual who has had massive weight loss, despite the long incisions that span most of the circum-ference of the upper body. Although extensive scars on the upper body are more difficult to conceal, this may be an acceptable trade-off for obtaining dramatic improvement in upper body shape.

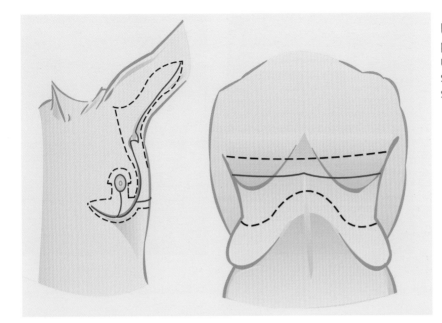

Upper Body Lift. Incision placement, front and back, for an upper body lift, which includes skin removal from the upper back, sides, breasts, and arms.

UNDERGOING AN UPPER BODY LIFT

With the patient under general anesthesia, the surgeon typically begins by doing a breast lift. The incision is made along the natural crease at the base of each breast and extends onto each side of the chest. In cases where extreme amounts of skin are being removed from the sides and the back, the incision may extend all the way across the back. In these cases, the incision is kept within what would be considered a woman's "bra line." In some cases, the incision may be extended towards the underarm and continued as an arm lift incision.

Once excess skin and fat are removed, incisions are closed and several drains are inserted. Some surgeons may place a compression garment over your upper body for a period of time to help resolve swelling and to provide support until your incisions heal. An upper body lift can take four to six hours to complete.

AFTER UPPER BODY LIFT SURGERY

Following upper body lift surgery, you will likely spend one to two days in the hospital, and require medication for mild to moderate pain. Following discharge from the hospital, you will return to the surgeon's

Questions to Ask Your Surgeon

- What are my options for arm contouring?
- Would staging procedures be a better option to obtain the best result?
- What are my options for chest contouring?
- Can any of these procedures be combined?
- Where will the scars be located?
- Will I be in a compression garment? For how long?
- What are the risks of surgery?
- What type of anesthesia do you recommend?
- When can I return to work?

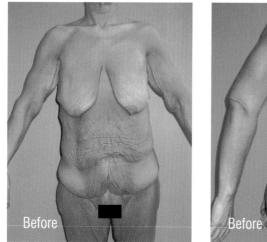
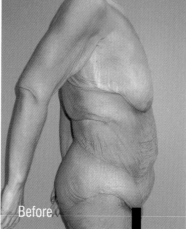
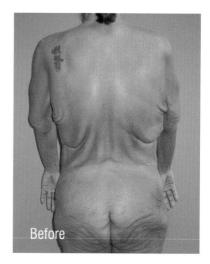

Age: 39. Weight lost: 210 pounds after gastric bypass

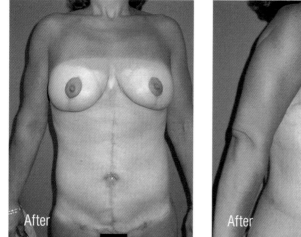
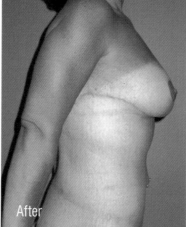
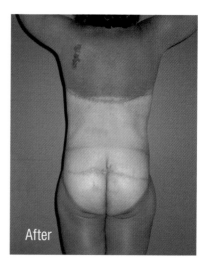

Procedure: upper body lift and breast lift
Postoperative: 6 months. Preoperative BMI: 27

office in two to five days to have the dressings and drains removed. It is important to wear the postoperative compression garment as instructed. If an arm lift is part of your upper body lift procedure, it is important to follow the precautions outlined previously. In most cases, following upper body lift surgery, you will be able to return to light duty work in two to four weeks and resume strenuous activity in four to six weeks.

RISKS OF ARM, CHEST, AND UPPER BODY LIFTS

Abnormal Scar Formation: Hypertrophic scars and keloids may form with greater frequency on the chest and arms.

Tissue Edema: Tissue swelling in the arms may persist or become chronic.

Wound Separation: Small areas of the wound may open up, in particular along the brachioplasty incision at the armpit or axilla.

Recurrent Laxity: Due to the weaker tissue quality along the inner arm, recurrent skin looseness occurs with a greater frequency.

Upper Body Contouring Surgery

Length of Surgery:	Arm lift and male breast reduction procedures 2 to 3 hours; upper body lift 4 to 6 hours
Type of Anesthesia:	General
Number of Drains:	2 to 4, usually removed within 2 to 5 days
Bandages:	Removed in 2 to 5 days
Sutures:	Usually none to be removed
Swelling:	75% resolved by 6 weeks; up to 1 year for complete resolution. Slower resolution for the upper arms
Duration of Hospital Stay:	1 to 2 days for upper body lift
Pain Level:	Mild to moderate
Back to Work:	1 to 2 weeks arm lift, male breast reduction, light duty; 2 to 4 weeks upper body lift, light duty
Activity Restriction:	No heavy lifting or strenuous activity for 4 to 6 weeks
Fully Mature Scars:	12 to 18 months
Final Contour Result:	6 to 12 months

CHAPTER 12

Face Lifts and Neck Lifts

Losing a great deal of weight can bring dramatic changes to your face and neck. Fortunately, these areas are less subject to the extreme degrees of skin excess that may be found elsewhere on the body. Furthermore, these changes are unlikely to result in significant health or functional problems. Nevertheless, skin excess and sagging in the face and neck are not as easily hidden and may significantly impact your self-esteem and self-image. You may view rejuvenating your face and neck as another step in creating a more youthful, refreshed appearance.

WHAT IS A FACE LIFT?

A face lift rejuvenates the lower two-thirds of the face by tightening loose skin and underlying muscles. Because excess skin is pulled back and trimmed off, a face lift can also smooth wrinkles and creases in the skin. A face lift, known in medical terms as a *rhytidectomy*, can give your face a more youthful, less tired appearance.

There are probably more ways to perform a face lift than any other plastic surgery procedure. However, the most useful and commonly performed face lift after massive weight loss is the standard face lift. This type of face lift also tightens the curtain of muscle just below the facial skin. This muscle is the SMAS layer, which refers to the *subcutaneous musculo-aponeurotic system*. Why is tightening these muscles important? Because they begin to sag as part of the aging process. By tightening this muscle layer, the face lift lasts longer and the skin is smoothed more naturally, avoiding a pulled look.

WHAT IS A NECK LIFT?

A neck lift procedure, known as a *cervicoplasty*, gives greater definition to the angle between the jawline and the neck by removing loose skin. In the majority of cases, a neck lift is performed as part of a face lift procedure. In fact, when a lot of skin excess is present in the neck, it is not possible to provide an adequate lift without using the incision required for a face lift procedure. In most cases, the surgeon also makes a small incision under the chin, through which fat can be suctioned and the thin muscle covering the neck can be tightened. This part of the surgery, involving the incision under the chin, is called a *submentoplasty*.

117

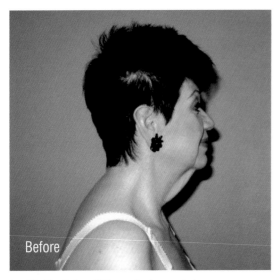

Before

Age 55. Weight lost: 150 pounds after gastric bypass

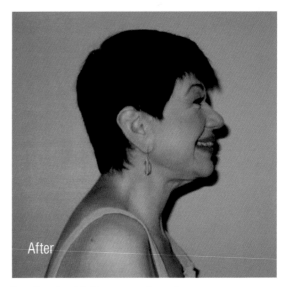

After

Procedure: face lift. Postoperative 8 months
Preoperative BMI: 31

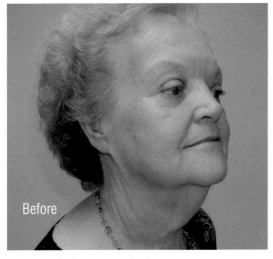

Before

Age 63. Weight lost: 135 pounds after gastric bypss

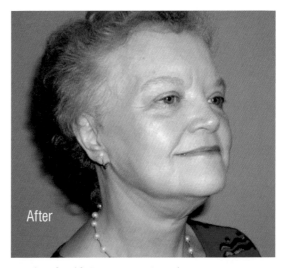

After

Procedure: face lift. Postoperative: 6 months
Preoperative BMI: 31

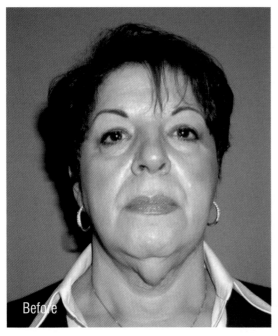

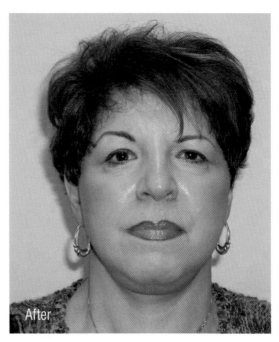

Age: 50. 100 pounds after gastric bypass

Procedure: face lift. Six months postoperative
Preoperative BMI: 43

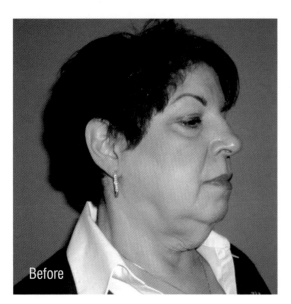

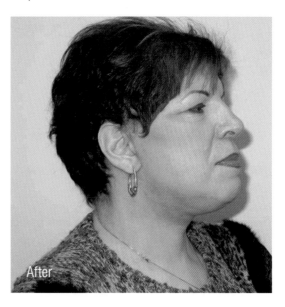

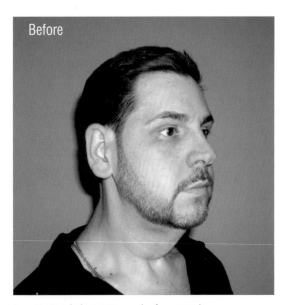

Before

After

Age: 35. Weight lost: 178 pounds after gastric bypass

Procedure: face lift. Postoperative: 4 months
Preoperative BMI: 34

The Male Neck Lift

For men who wish to avoid a face lift procedure, there is a unique type of neck lift procedure that directly excises excess skin in the neck. This leaves a substantial scar that runs down the center of the neck and is shaped in the form of the letter "Z". However, in men this scar typically blends well with the surrounding skin and can be covered with a beard. For women, a scar in this area can be quite noticeable; there is also a greater risk for abnormal scar formation due to different skin characteristics between men and women. Some men may not object to a visible scar on the neck; they may however object to changing their looks with a face lift procedure, which can alter the hairline and sideburns. Recovery following this type of neck lift is also substantially less than that after face lift surgery.

INSURANCE CONSIDERATIONS

In general, face and neck contouring procedures are considered cosmetic in nature and do not qualify for insurance coverage.

UNDERGOING FACE AND NECK CONTOURING SURGERY

If you're having face and neck contouring surgery, you may be given either intravenous sedation or general anesthesia. The neck lift is usually performed first. Often, this involves liposuction to remove fatty deposits in the neck. An incision below the chin allows access to the *platysma*, a thin sheet of muscle that covers the neck area. Tightening this muscle with sutures provides for a smoother neck contour.

To begin the face lift procedure, an incision is made behind the hairline in the temple area; this incision extends down the "sideburn" in front of the ear, under the earlobe and into the scalp area in the neck. The skin is lifted and fat is trimmed away or suctioned. The surgeon will then tighten the SMAS layer. The skin is redraped and the excess is trimmed away.

At the end of the procedure, a surgical drain is usually placed on each side of the face. A soft bulky dressing is then used to wrap the head and cover the wounds. The face lift procedure will take three to four hours to complete.

AFTER YOUR SURGERY

Following a face lift procedure you are usually monitored overnight in an outpatient facility for signs of bleeding. Your face

will feel tight due to normal swelling. The application of cold compresses will help speed healing. Postoperative pain from a face lift procedure is usually mild. For the first twenty-four hours after a face or neck lift, minimize chewing, talking and other activities that require facial movements. When you sleep, you'll need to keep your head elevated—propped up with pillows—to minimize swelling. In most cases, any drains that were placed will be removed prior to your going home.

RECOVERING AT HOME

It is important for you to carefully follow your surgeon's postoperative instructions. You will return to your doctor's office two to five days after surgery to have the dressings removed and the incisions checked. Sutures and skin staples that are

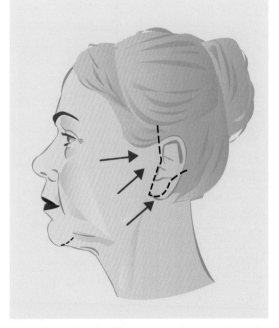

Incisions for standard face lift; arrows show direction of skin pull.

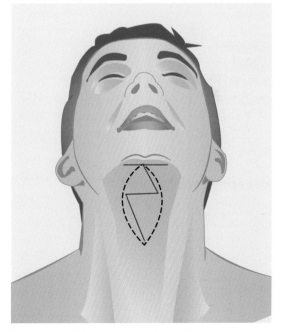

Direct excision of skin excess in a male neck lift

121

placed behind the ears are typically removed in five to ten days. Although you may be able to return to work within one to two weeks, this will depend on how comfortable you are with bruising and swelling that is likely still present. Make-up can usually provide adequate camouflage and can be applied after seven to ten days.

Skin numbness can be expected to last for several weeks. Although there will be significant resolution in swelling by two to three weeks, it will take two to three months to see the final results of your facial contouring surgery.

SPECIAL CONSIDERATIONS

Treating Skin Quality

Although a face lift procedure will soften deep furrows or creases in the skin, it will not adequately treat finer wrinkles that may be present. This requires *skin resurfacing*, which can be performed with a chemical peel, dermabrasion or laser resurfacing. Injection of botulinum toxin, known as Botox, can also weaken facial muscles that produce these wrinkles and provide improvement, although only on a temporary basis. Depending on the nature of the wrinkle, temporary fillers can also be injected to soften the line.

Restoring Facial Volume

Although a face lift procedure will lift and re-drape skin and underlying tissues to a more youthful position, it will not fully restore volume. To provide greater fullness, there are a number of options to consider, including soft tissue fillers, sometimes called "wrinkle fillers." These include such agents as collagen, Restylane and Sculptra; your own body fat may also be used in some

cases. Silicone implants may be an option for augmenting the cheeks or the chin.

Maintaining Balance

In addition to performing a face lift procedure, upper and lower eyelid lifts (*blepharoplasty*) and a *forehead lift* will provide for a more balanced and rejuvenated look.

Often, these procedures are performed along with a face lift procedure. You can explore these options further with your plastic surgeon.

Face and Neck Contouring Surgery

Length of Surgery:	3 to 4 hours
Length of Stay:	Outpatient overnight stay
Type of Anesthesia:	Intravenous sedation or general
Number of Drains:	May have one on each side of the face, removed in 24 hours
Bandages:	Removed in 1 to 2 days
Sutures:	Removed in 5 to 10 days Skin staples behind the ear removed with little discomfort
Swelling:	Significant resolution by 2 to 3 weeks
Pain Level:	Mild
Back to Work:	1 to 2 weeks
Activity Restriction:	No heavy lifting or strenuous activity for 3 to 4 weeks
Fully Mature Scars:	12 to 18 months
Final Contour Result:	2 to 3 months

RISKS OF FACE LIFT AND NECK LIFT SURGERY

Hematoma: A collection of blood that occurs following surgery and can lead to a dangerous reduction in circulation to the skin. This may require a trip back to the operating room to remove the blood and to control any ongoing bleeding. In general, this risk is higher in men. Other factors that can significantly increase this risk include uncontrolled high blood pressure and blood thinning medications such as aspirin (See Appendix E).

Necrosis (Skin Death): This results from loss of circulation to the skin and can lead to loss of skin, often behind or just in front of the ear. This can significantly delay wound healing and may lead to a highly visible scar. Smokers have a much higher risk for this complication to occur.

Nerve Injury: Injury to nerves can lead to numbness of the ear or muscle paralysis in the face with asymmetry and change in facial expression. Nerve function may require months to recover. Permanent nerve injury is uncommon.

TIPS FOR RECOVERY

- If you smoke, you must stop smoking for at least four weeks before and after your surgery to minimize the risk for complications and to allow your skin to heal properly.

- Allowing sideburns to grow out before surgery will help camouflage the scar.

- Have mouthwash available since it may be several days until you will be able to fully brush your teeth.

- Avoid sun exposure to your incision sites for as long as the scars are still red. Sun exposure will result in darkening with a more conspicuous scar. If you must expose these areas to the sun, apply a sunscreen with a sun protection factor (SPF) of 30 or higher.

- Flexible straws will make drinking liquids easier.

- Have a telephone with a speakerphone available next to your bed.

- Lubricating eye drops will help with dry eyes which may result from anesthesia.

- Frozen peas placed in a plastic bag can serve effectively as an ice pack to reduce postoperative swelling.

Questions to Ask Your Surgeon

- What are my options for contouring of the face and neck?
- What type of face lift do you recommend?
- Where will the scars be located?
- How will a face lift procedure affect the appearance of my hairline and sideburns?
- Am I a candidate for other facial rejuvenating procedures?
- What are the risks of surgery?

123

Closing Remarks

You have traveled a long and difficult road to achieve your new look. You have taken pounds and inches off your body. You have changed your lifestyle and adopted new habits for healthier living, from increasing your activity levels to modifying your eating patterns. You are to be applauded not only for making a commitment to get healthy and look your best, but also for sticking to that commitment.

YOUR FEELINGS AND SELF-IMAGE

It may be easier to adapt to your new body on the physical level than on the emotional one. The psychology behind how each of us sees ourselves is a complex matter.

After body contouring, don't be surprised if you experience conflicting emotions at first. You may feel happy with your body one day, sad about your scars the next. Some days you may feel overwhelmed by the amazing changes you've undergone. If you have been overweight for much of your life, you may have a difficult time now regarding yourself as someone of average or normal weight. You may still feel overweight even though you aren't.

Once these up and down feelings settle, you should enjoy greater self-confidence. But if you still find yourself struggling with your feelings over time, talking with a counselor or sharing your feelings in a support group may be of great help to you. Remember: Many other people have walked in your shoes. You don't need to be a superman or superwoman and go through this emotional journey alone. Sharing your story with others who have had similar experiences, and hearing about their struggles and triumphs, can give you the moral support needed to keep you on track.

If you have been suffering from depression, understand that body contouring is not a treatment for a depressive disorder. Your new appearance and newfound freedom certainly may alleviate symptoms of depression, but seek professional treatment if you continue to experience debilitating depression. Treatment may involve taking antidepressant medications, but many people improve greatly from counseling alone.

Despite any conflicting feelings after body contouring, ultimately you can expect your self-confidence and self-image to improve. By far, individuals who have had body contouring surgery are thankful to be able to lead a normal, active life, unencumbered by physical limitations that previously held them back. Being able to do what you love to do, keeping stress levels down, and creating a positive environment go a long way in helping you lead a healthy and positive life.

EXPECT CHANGES IN RELATIONSHIPS

Changes in relationship dynamics are common after major weight loss and body contouring surgery. Some of your friends may not be able to adapt to your physical and lifestyle transformations, and they may eventually become less prominent in your life. At the same time, your more active lifestyle and changing priorities will create opportunities for new people to come into your life. You will probably make new friends who are drawn to your higher levels of energy and enthusiasm.

Your relationship with your mate may change as well, for better or worse. Your relationship may improve, with both of you enjoying a fresh new start and embracing new opportunities that come your way. Or, you may choose to go your separate ways. Everybody handles change differently.

LIVING LIFE TO THE FULLEST

You have invested a great deal into improving your body—not only your time and money but also your energy, hard work, hopes, and dreams. With so much focus on your physical being, don't forget that you are so much more than your body. You have people in your life whom you love and who love you. You have dreams, goals, careers, and personal interests. All of these give your life great depth and dimension. You have a unique personality and the ability to love, learn, and enjoy life. As important and miraculous as your body is, don't forget about the rest of you—your emotions, your passion, your purpose, your soul, and your spirit. Let your new body serve as the vehicle to facilitate living your life to the fullest.

APPENDIX A

Body Mass Index Table

Height (inches)	Normal						Overweight					Obese										Extreme Obesity															
BMI	19	20	21	22	23	24	25	26	27	28	29	30	31	32	33	34	35	36	37	38	39	40	41	42	43	44	45	46	47	48	49	50	51	52	53	54
												Body Weight (pounds)																								
58	91	96	100	105	110	115	119	124	129	134	138	143	148	153	158	162	167	172	177	181	186	191	196	201	205	210	215	220	224	229	234	239	244	248	253	258
59	94	99	104	109	114	119	124	128	133	138	143	148	153	158	163	168	173	178	183	188	193	198	203	208	212	217	222	227	232	237	242	247	252	257	262	267
60	97	102	107	112	118	123	128	133	138	143	148	153	158	163	168	174	179	184	189	194	199	204	209	215	220	225	230	235	240	245	250	255	261	266	271	276
61	100	106	111	116	122	127	132	137	143	148	153	158	164	169	174	180	185	190	195	201	206	211	217	222	227	232	238	243	248	254	259	264	269	275	280	285
62	104	109	115	120	126	131	136	142	147	153	158	164	169	175	180	186	191	196	202	207	213	218	224	229	235	240	246	251	256	262	267	273	278	284	289	295
63	107	113	118	124	130	135	141	146	152	158	163	169	175	180	186	191	197	203	208	214	220	225	231	237	242	248	254	259	265	270	278	282	287	293	299	304
64	110	116	122	128	134	140	145	151	157	163	169	174	180	186	192	197	204	209	215	221	227	232	238	244	250	256	262	267	273	279	285	291	296	302	308	314
65	114	120	126	132	138	144	150	156	162	168	174	180	186	192	198	204	210	216	222	228	234	240	246	252	258	264	270	276	282	288	294	300	306	312	318	324
66	118	124	130	136	142	148	155	161	167	173	179	186	192	198	204	210	216	223	229	235	241	247	253	260	266	272	278	284	291	297	303	309	315	322	328	334
67	121	127	134	140	146	153	159	166	172	178	185	191	198	204	211	217	223	230	236	242	249	255	261	268	274	280	287	293	299	306	312	319	325	331	338	344
68	125	131	138	144	151	158	164	171	177	184	190	197	203	210	216	223	230	236	243	249	256	262	269	276	282	289	295	302	308	315	322	328	335	341	348	354
69	128	135	142	149	155	162	169	176	182	189	196	203	209	216	223	230	236	243	250	257	263	270	277	284	291	297	304	311	318	324	331	338	345	351	358	365
70	132	139	146	153	160	167	174	181	188	195	202	209	216	222	229	236	243	250	257	264	271	278	285	292	299	306	313	320	327	334	341	348	355	362	369	376
71	136	143	150	157	165	172	179	186	193	200	208	215	222	229	236	243	250	257	265	272	279	286	293	301	308	315	322	329	338	343	351	358	365	372	379	386
72	140	147	154	162	169	177	184	191	199	206	213	221	228	235	242	250	258	265	272	279	287	294	302	309	316	324	331	338	346	353	361	368	375	383	390	397
73	144	151	159	166	174	182	189	197	204	212	219	227	235	242	250	257	265	272	280	288	295	302	310	318	325	333	340	348	355	363	371	378	386	393	401	408
74	148	155	163	171	179	186	194	202	210	218	225	233	241	249	256	264	272	280	287	295	303	311	319	326	334	342	350	358	365	373	381	389	396	404	412	420
75	152	160	168	176	184	192	200	208	216	224	232	240	248	256	264	272	279	287	295	303	311	319	327	335	343	351	359	367	375	383	391	399	407	415	423	431
76	156	164	172	180	189	197	205	213	221	230	238	246	254	263	271	279	287	295	304	312	320	328	336	344	353	361	369	377	385	394	402	410	418	426	435	443

Source: Adapted from *Clinical Guidelines on the Identification, Evaluation, and Treatment of Overweight and Obesity in Adults: The Evidence Report*.

Weight Loss Surgery Procedures

Bariatric (from the Greek word *baros* for weight) surgery, also known as obesity or weight-loss surgery, is performed on the stomach and intestines in morbidly obese individuals who have failed all other methods of weight loss. By definition, morbidly obese individuals have a high body mass index (BMI) of at least 40, which in the average adult equates to being roughly one hundred pounds overweight. Some individuals with a lower BMI and serious obesity-related health problems may also qualify.

TYPES OF WEIGHT-LOSS SURGERY

Bariatric surgery has evolved since the early 1950s to its present-day form, which includes several different procedures, all of which share the goal of modifying dietary habits that will aid in long-term weight maintenance. Weight loss through surgery can be achieved by either restricting the amount of food that can be ingested or in combination with altering the manner in which food is processed and absorbed. The procedures used today therefore fall into two broad categories: combined restrictive-malabsorptive and restrictive procedures.

Combined Restrictive-Malabsorptive Procedures

These procedures combine the restriction of food intake with malabsorption of nutrients to varying degrees. They typically require lifelong replacement of certain vitamins and minerals to avoid serious nutritional deficiencies.

Gastric Bypass: Also known as the RYGB, RGB, or Roux-en-Y Gastric Bypass, it is the most widely recognized bariatric procedure. It is the most common procedure performed in the United States today, and is the gold standard by which results from other procedures are measured. Through stapling, the stomach is typically reduced to the size of your thumb, which greatly restricts food intake. The food that exits this new stomach is then bypassed to a more distant portion of the small intestine.

Since the small intestine is where the absorption of food takes place, this results in a malabsorption of nutrients, and a consequent decreased absorption of calories. *Dumping syndrome* is common. This results from the rapid transit of foods high in sugar into the small bowel, with unpleasant side effects such as abdominal cramping, dizziness, palpitations, nausea, sweating and faintness. Long-term results with the gastric bypass are typically show a loss of 70 percent of excess weight.

Biliopancreatic Diversion (BPD): This procedure also utilizes stapling to reduce the size of the stomach, although not to the same degree as in the gastric bypass. The effectiveness of this procedure lies in the greater utilization of malabsorption. The digestive enzymes necessary for food absorption are diverted to a point much further downstream in the small intestine. This results in a more significant malabsorption of nutrients and associated calories. Although results are impressive at near 80 percent loss of excess weight, the risk for nutritional and metabolic complications increases significantly in comparison to the gastric bypass. Often, this procedure is reserved for the superobese individual with a BMI of at least 50. Severe malnutrition or protein deficiency is a risk.

Duodenal Switch (DS): This is essentially the biliopancreatic diversion with several important modifications. The stomach is reduced to a greater degree, although in such a manner as to allow greater absorption of Vitamin B_{12}, as well as to reduce the incidence of dumping syndrome and ulcer formation. The degree of malabsorption is slightly less; therefore more protein can be absorbed. Nevertheless, the risk for nutritional and metabolic complications is still significant.

Long-Limb Gastric Bypass (LLGB): Also known as the distal gastric bypass or very long-limb gastric bypass, this procedure modifies the gastric bypass through greater utilization of malabsorption by preventing the digestion of food until much further downstream. Similar to the biliopancreatic diversion, the risk for significant nutritional deficiencies is greater and this procedure is therefore often reserved for the superobese individual.

Mini-Gastric Bypass: Typically performed laparoscopically, this procedure is similar to standard gastric bypass, with the main difference being the use of a "loop" configuration to attach the intestine to the new stomach pouch, instead of the Roux-en-Y configuration. Although technically simpler to perform, this procedure can result in significant reflux of bile into the esophagus, causing irritation and ulcer formation, with an increased risk for esophageal cancer. This procedure is therefore not widely accepted.

Banded Gastric Bypass: This is a gastric-bypass procedure that includes the use of a synthetic band placed around the opening of the new stomach pouch. This band may limit future stretching and widening of the pouch outlet, thereby preventing the passage of larger amounts of food into the intestine.

Restrictive Procedures

Restrictive procedures focus primarily on restricting the amount of food that can be ingested. They were developed to avoid the sometimes serious nutritional complications that can accompany procedures utilizing malabsorption. These surgeries modify the stomach only and do not alter the anatomy of the small intestine. Lifelong nutritional supplementation is usually not required.

Vertical Banded Gastroplasty (VBG): Through stapling, a small stomach pouch is created, the outlet of which is then restricted with placement of a rigid band. The narrow outlet forces food to stay in the pouch longer, making you feel full more quickly and giving you the sensation of being full for a longer period of time. Lacking a malabsorptive component, results are in the range of 40 to 50 percent loss of excess weight.

Laparoscopic Adjustable Gastric Band (LAGB): This is among the least invasive of procedures, and is rapidly gaining in popularity. Performed laparoscopically, an adjustable silicone band is placed around the top of the stomach, where food enters from the esophagus. There is a small balloon on the inner surface of the band, connected by tubing to an access port placed outside the abdomen, under the skin. By accessing the port with a needle, the balloon can be filled with saline, thereby further narrowing the band and restricting food intake. There is no stapling or division of the stomach. One advantage is long-term adjustability. The band can also be loosened or "reversed" at any time, such as during pregnancy when food restriction could be harmful to the fetus. This procedure also carries minimal risk for serious complications. At present, the only adjustable gastric band on the U.S. market that is FDA-approved is the LAP-BAND. To be successful, this procedure does require strict commitment to dietary recommendations and regular follow-up for adjustment. Weight loss is much slower compared to the gastric-bypass procedure.

LAPAROSCOPIC VERSUS OPEN PROCEDURES

Laparoscopic or minimally invasive surgery involves the use of a small camera to perform surgery through five to six small incisions, ranging from five to twelve millimeters in length. Following the first laparoscopic gastric bypass in the early 1990s, the field of bariatric surgery has been revolutionized by this approach. There is a significant benefit both in terms of the reduction of wound complications, such as infection and hernia formation, as well as a faster recovery with less discomfort.

One disadvantage of laparoscopy, however, is a significantly higher incidence of intestinal obstruction than with open gastric-bypass procedures. Although nearly every bariatric procedure can be performed laparoscopically, the vast majority are laparoscopic gastric bypass and LAP-BAND procedures.

OTHER PROCEDURES

Although not entirely a new concept, the placement of a gastric or stomach pacemaker to control food intake is receiving greater attention. As technology is refined, and in combination with the laparoscopic approach, this may prove to be effective and even less invasive than the LAP-BAND procedure. There have also been trials with an intragastric balloon, which takes up space in the stomach and causes the feeling of fullness soon after eating. However, weight-loss results have not been impressive with this procedure and the level of potentially severe complications is high.

APPENDIX
C

Nutrition

Malnutrition can develop following any surgical weight loss procedure. Bariatric surgery alters the way food and its nutrients are processed by the body for digestion. Often, there is a component of malabsorption, in which nutrients that are taken in by mouth are not fully absorbed by the intestine. Nutritional deficiencies following bariatric surgery frequently develop from a combination of malabsorption and intolerance to certain foods that contain important nutrients.

Deficiencies of vitamins, minerals and protein are relatively common and may lead to complications with body contouring surgery. In many cases, conditions related to malnutrition may not become apparent until one or more years following weight-loss surgery. Some of these nutritional deficiencies can also develop following non-surgical weight loss using very restricted diets, especially if weight loss is rapid or significant.

Bariatric Procedure	Most Common Deficiencies
Gastric Bypass	Vitamin B12, Folate, Calcium, Iron
Malabsorptive Procedures: Biliopancreatic Diversion, Duodenal Switch, Long-limb and Distal Gastric Bypass	Protein, Calcium, Iron, Fat-soluble Vitamins (Vitamins A,D,E and K)
Restrictive Procedures*: Lap-BAND, Vertical Banded Gastroplasty	Thiamin, Potassium, Folate

*Although absorption of nutrients is normal, deficiency may develop from persistent vomiting or suboptimal/reduced nutritional intake.

Nutrient	Recommended Dietary Allowance (RDA)	Deficiency	Important Food Sources
Vitamin B$_{12}$	2.4 microgram/day	Anemia, weakness, numbness in extremities, coma, permanent neurological damage	Eggs, dairy, fish, red meat, shellfish
Iron	8.0-18 milligram/day	Anemia, fatigue, headache, brittle fingernails, impaired immune system	Red meat, shellfish, lima beans, prune juice
Folate (Folic Acid)	400 microgram/day	Anemia, diarrhea, fatigue	Leafy greens, fruits, meats, eggs, lima beans
Calcium	1000-1200 milligram/day*	Bone loss (osteoporosis), bone pain, numbness, diarrhea	Dairy products, tofu, almonds
Thiamin (vitamin B$_1$)	1.1-1.2 milligram/day	Weakness, numbness in extremities, coma, permanent neurological damage	Fortified whole-grain products, cereals, legumes
Zinc	8-11 milligram/day	Wound healing difficulty, hair loss, depressed immune function, rash	Red meat, poultry, oysters, beans
Vitamin A	700-900 microgram/day	Night blindness, dry eyes, rash	Eggs, milk, liver, carrots
Vitamin D	5-10 microgram/day*	Osteomalacia, bone pain, muscle weakness	Cod liver oil, fortified milk, salmon, tuna
Vitamin E	15 milligram/day	Weakness, anemia, eczema, poor concentration	Leafy greens, nuts, vegetable oil
Vitamin K	90-120 microgram/day	Impaired blood clotting	Leafy greens, tree fruits
Magnesium	310-420 milligram/day	Muscle cramps, weakness, abnormal heartbeat, seizures	Leafy greens, legumes, nuts, fish
Potassium	4.7 gram/day	Muscle weakness, abnormal heartbeat, confusion	Fruits, vegetables, nuts, legumes
Protein	46-56 gram/day	Wound healing difficulty, anemia, hair loss, depressed immune function, tissue edema	Beef, poultry, fish, eggs, milk, cheese, yogurt
Total Water [a]	2.7-3.7 liter/day	Low blood pressure, weakness, risk for blood clots, kidney stones, urinary tract infection	All beverages, moisture in food

[a]Total water contained in food, beverages and drinking water.
* Represents Adequate Intake (AI).
Source: The National Academy of Sciences.

Nutritional deficiencies following bariatric surgery can usually be prevented or corrected with dietary supplementation. For this reason, regular long-term follow-up with a bariatric dietician is important. Although the RDA values listed above are for healthy individuals and do not factor in malabsorption or rapid weight loss, they nevertheless set minimum nutritional requirements that, if met, will prevent a large number of deficiencies after weight loss surgery.

The following are guidelines regarding specific nutrients. Importantly, you must follow specific recommendations regarding your nutrition and dietary supplementation given by your bariatric surgeon, dietician and plastic surgeon. Their recommendations will be based on nutritional requirements specific to your procedure as well as the results from laboratory tests and regular follow-up evaluation.

IMPORTANT DIETARY SUPPLEMENTS:

Protein

Regardless of the method of weight loss, protein must be adequately replenished. Dietary protein is broken down into amino acids in the intestine, nine of which are indispensable or essential amino acids which cannot be produced by the body. Dietary protein must therefore be of high quality, such as animal protein, which contains these indispensable amino acids. Following bariatric surgery, a minimum of 60 grams of protein per day or 0.8 to 1.5 grams of protein per kilogram of lean body mass is usually required. These requirements may increase to 90 grams per day or more following malabsorptive procedures. Often, protein shakes are used to fulfill

these requirements during the rapid weight loss phase, and these may also be recommended by your plastic surgeon following major body contouring procedures when protein requirements for healing wounds are high.

Multivitamin

Daily lifelong supplementation with one to two multivitamins is a minimum requirement following gastric bypass or malabsorptive procedures. This should be a high potency adult multivitamin or prenatal multivitamin.

Vitamin B$_{12}$ and Folate

In addition to malabsorption, there may be an intolerance to foods that are an important source of vitamin B$_{12}$ and folate. Deficiencies in vitamin B$_{12}$ and folate are fairly common following bariatric operations. Although oral supplementation of at least 350 micrograms of vitamin B$_{12}$ per day is adequate, following gastric bypass, vitamin B$_{12}$ is best taken by injection (1000 micrograms every month for the first year and then every 2 to 3 months thereafter) or sublingually (special formulation placed beneath the tongue). A multivitamin with a folate content of at least 400 micrograms is usually adequate to prevent deficiency.

Iron and Calcium

Menstruating women are at greatest risk for developing anemia from iron deficiency. Often, they are treated prophylactically with iron supplementation. Iron deficiency, if present, is usually treated with an oral supplement containing elemental iron (180 to 220 milligrams/day). Iron should be taken together with chewable vitamin C (500mg) or citrus juice (orange or grapefruit juice) to help with absorption. There are also iron supplements that contain vitamin C. A stool softener or mild laxative will help avoid constipation common with iron supplementation.

Calcium deficiency may accelerate the development of osteoporosis. Calcium citrate is the preferred form for replacement with a daily dose in the range of 1200 to 1500 milligrams. Take calcium and iron at least one hour apart as they compete for absorption.

Vitamin A and D

Malabsorptive procedures carry the greatest risk for developing deficiency of the fat-soluble vitamins, which include A and D. Additional supplementation following procedures such as the biliopancreatic diversion is in the range of 25,000 to 50,000 IU daily for vitamin A and 10,000 to 50,000 IU weekly for vitamin D.

Water

Following bariatric surgery, there may be a limit on the amount of water that you can drink at one time, as well as restrictions on liquid intake at mealtime. Nevertheless, it is very important to drink enough water daily to prevent dehydration, which may increase the chance for a life-threatening blood clot following major body contouring surgery. Carrying and sipping from a water bottle containing a non-carbonated, caffeine-free and sugar-free beverage or plain water throughout the day will ensure adequate hydration.

Medications and Natural Supplements to Be Avoided Prior to Surgery

Medications listed below should be stopped 14 days prior to surgery with permission from your prescribing doctor. These medications could result in excessive bleeding, interact with anesthetic drugs or otherwise prevent proper healing. In addition, certain supplements and herbal remedies may have adverse effects. Any of these medications, supplements or herbal remedies that need to be continued should be cleared with your surgeon. In general, take Tylenol (acetaminophen) for pain relief.

Aspirin Medications to Avoid

4-Way Cold Tabs	5-Aminosalicylic Acid	Acetilsalicylic Acid
Adprin-B products	Alka-Seltzer products	Amigesic
Anacin products	Anexsia w/Codeine	Argesic-SA
Arthra-G	Arthriten products	Arthritis Foundation products
Arthritis Pain Formula	Arthritis Strength BC Powder	Arthropan
ASA	Asacol	Ascriptin products
Aspergum	Asprimox products	Axotal
Azdone	Azulfidine products	B-A-C
Backache Maximum Strength Relief	Bayer products	BC Powder
Bismatrol products	Buffered aspirin	Bufferin products
Buffetts 11	Buffex	Butal/ASA/Caff
Butalbital Compound	Cama Arthritis Pain Reliever	Carisoprodol Compound
Cheracol	Choline Magnesium Trisalicylate	Choline Salicylate

Aspirin Medications to Avoid (continued)

Damason-P	Darvon Compound-65	Darvon/ASA
Dipentum	Disalcid	Doan's products
Dolobid	Dristan	Duragesic
Easprin	Ecotrin products	Empirin products
Equagesic	Excedrin products	Fiorgen PF
Fiorinal products	Gelpirin	Genprin
Gensan	Goody's Extra Strength Headache Powders	Halfprin products
Isollyl Improved	Kaodene	Lanorinal
Lortab ASA	Magan	Magnaprin products
Magnesium Salicylate	Magsal	Marnal
Marthritic	Meprobamate	Mesalamine
Methocarbamol	Micrainin	Mobidin
Mobigesic	Momentum	Mono-Gesic
Night-Time Effervescent Cold	Norgesic products	Norwich products
Olsalazine	Orphengesic products	Oxycodone

Ibuprofen Medications to Avoid

Actron	Acular (opthalmic)	Advil products
Aleve	Anaprox products	Ansaid
Bayer Select	Cataflam	Clinoril
Celebrex	Daypro	Diclofenac
Dimetapp Sinus	Dristan Sinus	Etodolac
Feldene	Fenoprofen	Flurbiprofen
Genpril	Haltran	IBU
Ibuprin	Ibuprofen	Ibuprohm
Indochron E-R	Indocin products	Indomethacin products
Ketoprofen	Ketorolac	Lodine
Meclofenamate	Meclomen	Mefenamic Acid
Menadol	Midol products	Motrin products
Nabumetone	Nalfon products	Naprelan
Naprosyn products	Naprox X	Naproxen
Nuprin	Ocufen (opthalmic)	Orudis products
Oruvail	Oxaprozin	Piroxicam
Ponstel	Profenal	Relafen
Rhinocaps	Sine-Aid products	Sulindac
Suprofen	Tolectin products	Tolmetin
Toradol	Trendar	Vioxx
Voltaren		

Tricyclic Antidepressant Medications to Avoid

Adapin	Amitriptyline	Amoxapine
Anafranil	Asendin	Aventyl
Clomipramine	Desipramine	Doxepin
Elavil	Endep	Etrafon products
Imipramine	Janimine	Limbitrol products
Ludiomil	Maprotiline	Norpramin
Nortriptyline	Pamelor	Pertofrane
Protriptyline	Sinequan	Surmontil
Tofranil	Triavil	Trimipramine
Vivactil		

Other Medications to Avoid

4-Way w/ Codeine	A.C.A.	A-A Compound
Accutrim	Actifed	Anexsia
Anisindione	Anturane	Arthritis Bufferin
BC Tablets	Childrens Advil	Clinoril C
Contac	Coumadin	Dalteparin injection
Dicumerol	Dipyridamole	Doxycycline
Emagrin	Enoxaparin injection	Flagyl
Fragmin injection	Furadantin	Heparin
Heparin Hydrocortisone	Isollyl	Lovenox injection
Macrodantin Mellaril	Mellaril	Miradon
Opasal	Pan-PAC	Pentoxyfylline
Persantine	Phenylpropanolamine	Prednisone
Protamine	Pyrroxate	Ru-Tuss
Salatin	Sinex	Sofarin
Soltice	Sparine	Stelazine
Sulfinpyrazone	Tenuate	Tenuate Dospan
Thorazine	Ticlid	Ticlopidine
Trental	Ursinus	Vibramycin
Warfarin	Zyban	

Supplements and Herbal Remedies to Avoid

Ackee fruit	Alfalfa	Aloe
Argimony	Barley	Bilberry
Bitter melon	Burdock root	Carrot oil
Cayenne	Celery	Chamomile
Chromium	Coriander	Dandelion root
Devil's club	Dong Quai root	Echinacea
Eucalyptus	Fenugreek seeds	Feverfew
Fo-ti	Garlic	Ginger
Gingko	Gingko biloba	Ginseng
Gmena	Goldenseal	Gotu Kola
Grape seed	Green tea	Guarana
Guayusa	Hawthorn	Horse chestnut
Kava Kava	Lavender	Lemon verbena
Licorice Root	Ma Huang	Melatonin
Muwort	Nem seed oil	Onions
Papaya	Periwinkle	Selenium
St. John's Wort	Valerian/Valerian root	Vitamin E
Willow bark	Yellow root	Yohimbe

and reconstructive surgery, the society's mission is to advance quality care for plastic surgery patients. The ASPS Web site is informative, offering detailed explanations of surgical procedures and a plastic surgeon search feature.

American Hospital Directory

4350 Brownsboro Road
Suite 110
Louisville, KY 40207
Fax: 502-899-7738
www.ahd.com

A privately owned company, American Hospital Directory enables you to do a free online search for a hospital, by name or by geographical region. Detailed information is given for each hospital, including address and telephone number, Web site, statistics, type of facility, and available services.

Federation of State Medical Boards

P.O. Box 619850
Dallas, TX 75261-9850
Phone: 817-868-4000
Fax: 817-868-4099
www.fsmb.org
www.fsmb.org/directory_smb.html

This national organization is composed of 70 medical boards operating in the U.S., Guam, Puerto Rico, the U.S. Virgin Islands and the Commonwealth of the Northern Mariana Islands. The Federation's Web site provides a directory that lists individual boards to contact for specific information on physician licensing in your region.

Joint Commission on Accreditation of Healthcare Organizations

One Renaissance Blvd
Oakbrook Terrace, IL 60181
Phone: 630-792-5000
www.jcaho.org

A major accrediting organization, the JCAHO evaluates and accredits more than 15,000 healthcare organizations and programs in the United States. Its Web site's "General Public" section discusses a number of relevant topics including patient safety and preventing medication mistakes.

International Society of Aesthetic Plastic Surgery

45 Lyme Road #304
Hanover, NH 03755
Phone: 603-643-2325
Fax: 603-643-1444
www.isaps.org

A chapter of the global organization International Confederation for Plastic, Reconstructive and Aesthetic Surgery, ISAPS is the official entity and premier international forum for worldwide aesthetic plastic surgery. The Web site enables you to locate aesthetic plastic surgeons in more than 65 nations. The site's "Press Center" supplies global statistics about aesthetic plastic surgery procedures.

Obesity Action Coalition

4511 North Himes Avenue
Suite 250
Tampa, Florida 33614
Phone: 800-717-3117
www.obesityaction.org

The mission of the OAC is to educate patients, family members, and the public on obesity and morbid obesity. In addition, the OAC will increase obesity education, work to improve access to medical treatments for obese patients, advocate for safe and effective treatments and strive to eliminate the negative stigma associated with all types of obesity.

Obesity Help

Phone: 1-866-WLS-INFO (1-866-957-4636)
www.obesityhelp.com

This site was founded in 1998 to provide information, support, and assistance against discrimination for the millions of people who suffer from morbid obesity. At the Web site you'll find information on weight loss surgery as well as numerous online forums where community members discuss everything from obesity-related topics to general interest subjects.

Overeaters Anonymous

World Service Office
P.O. Box 44020
Rio Rancho, NM 87174-4020
Phone: 505-891-2664
Fax: 505-891-4320
www.oa.org

This 12-step program of recovery from compulsive overeating holds meetings worldwide and offers tools to help individuals refrain from compulsive eating. The Web site enables you to find a meeting in your area.

Society for Nutrition Education (SNE)

7150 Winton Drive
Suite 300
Indianapolis, IN 46268
(317) 328-4627 or (800) 235-6690
(317) 280-8527
www.sne.org

SNE represents the professional interests of nutrition educators by educating and influencing policy makers about nutrition, food, and health.

Glossary

abdominal cavity: the region inside the abdomen that holds the stomach and other organs.

abdominal wall: a wall comprised of muscle, connective tissue, fat and skin that encloses the abdominal cavity.

abdominoplasty: a tummy tuck or abdominal contouring procedure.

abdominoplasty, anchor: a modified tummy tuck procedure with a vertical incision down the middle of the abdomen in addition to the standard lower horizontal incision, which results in an anchor-shaped scar.

abdominoplasty, endoscopic: a tummy tuck procedure performed through a small incision with the aid of a specialized camera, and used primarily for correction of rectus diastasis.

abdominoplasty, extended: a modified tummy tuck procedure in which the incision extends around the waistline and onto the back area.

abdominoplasty, fleur-de-lis: same as anchor abdominoplasty.

abdominoplasty, full: the most common tummy tuck procedure with an incision extending from hip bone to hip bone, in which excess skin and fat is removed and there is correction of rectus diastasis.

abdominoplasty, high-lateral-tension: a modified tummy tuck procedure in which greater emphasis is placed on pulling the tissue tighter along the outer part of the abdomen.

abdominoplasty, mini: a partial tummy tuck procedure in which the incision is short and primarily effective for removing excess skin below the level of the belly button.

abdominoplasty, reverse: an abdominal contouring procedure in which the incision is made at the top of the abdomen, usually in the breast crease, with upward pull to remove excess skin and fat primarily along the upper portion of the abdomen.

abdominoplasty, standard: same as full abdominoplasty.

abdominoplasty, upper: same as reverse abdominoplasty.

abscess: collection of pus or infected fluid.

absorbable sutures: surgical stitches that dissolve on their own after a period of time and do not need to be removed by a doctor.

adequate intake (AI): a recommended average daily intake for a particular nutrient when the RDA cannot be determined.

adipose: pertaining to fat.

adjustable gastric band: a surgical weight loss procedure in which an adjustable band is placed around the neck of the stomach to restrict food intake.

adrenaline: a naturally occurring hormone which acts as a stimulant.

aesthetic surgery: cosmetic surgery.

albumin: a protein found in the body, used to assess nutritional status.

ambulatory surgery center (ASC): a facility where surgical procedures are performed and the patient is released the same day.

American Board of Plastic Surgery (ABPS): the major specialty board responsible for certifying plastic and reconstructive surgeons.

amino acids: the basic building blocks of protein.

amnestic effect: partial or total loss of memory of events surrounding the administration of certain drugs used for anesthesia.

anabolism: the phase of metabolism in which complex materials of living tissues are made.

analgesics: prescription or nonprescription drugs that relieve pain.

android body type: apple-shaped figure.

anemia: a low blood count.

anesthesiologist: a physician trained to administer anesthesia.

antibiotics: medication used to treat or prevent infection.

areola: the circular pigmented area surrounding the nipple of the breast.

arm lift: a surgical procedure that removes excess skin, and possibly excess fat, from the upper arms and tightens the inner tissue to improve the shape of the arm.

arrhythmia: abnormal heart rhythm.

aspiration pneumonia: the inhalation of fluid from the stomach into the lungs, causing pneumonia.

asthma: a respiratory disorder characterized by wheezing.

asymmetry: when two corresponding parts are unbalanced or disproportionate to each other.

atelectasis: incomplete expansion of the lungs.

augmentation: process of adding volume to specific body parts, typically the breasts or buttocks.

augmentation-mastopexy: a breast lift procedure combined with placement of a breast implant.

autoaugmentation: a surgical procedure that increases the size of a particular area such as the buttocks or the breasts with a patient's own tissue.

autologous fat graft: injection of fat obtained with liposuction from elsewhere on the body.

axilla: the armpit.

bariatric surgery: the surgical treatment of obesity.

bat wing deformity: extreme sagging of skin along the upper arms.

belt lipectomy: as initially described in 1960, the resection of excess tissue around the circumference of the torso. Combined with modern surgical technique, often referred to as a body lift procedure.

biliopancreatic diversion: a surgical weight loss procedure in which there is malabsorption of food.

bioelectrical impedance analysis (BIA): a method for estimating percent of body fat.

bleeding disorder: a condition in which bleeding is prolonged and excessive.

blepharoplasty: removal of excess skin and fat from the eyelids, upper or lower.

blood clot: a gelled mass of blood tissue.

blood transfusion: replacement of blood to treat anemia.

board certification: a status awarded by a professional association for a physician who has met specific standards of knowledge and clinical skills, usually by way of rigorous written and oral examination.

body contouring surgery: general term used to describe various surgical procedures done for cosmetic or reconstructive reasons.

body lift: a combination surgical procedure that contours the central body. Typically affects the abdomen, thighs, lower back, and buttocks.

body lift, central: another term for a body lift.

body lift, lower: a common term for body lift.

body lift, total: a true body lift combines upper and lower body contouring procedures to achieve total body restoration. However, the term is often used to refer to a lower body lift.

body lift, upper: a combination surgical procedure that incorporates several individual body contouring procedures to improve the upper body through one operation. Typically affects the upper back, sides, chest/breasts, and arms.

body mass index (BMI): a number that is calculated based on a person's height and weight, used to define the medical standard for obesity and gauge health risk factors.

Botox: the trade name for botulinum toxin type A.

botulinum toxin: a toxin which in diluted medical-grade form can be used to temporarily weaken facial muscles, thereby softening wrinkles.

bowel prep: a regimen for cleansing the colon with a laxative and antibiotics prior to surgery.

brachioplasty: arm lift.

brachioplasty, extended: a brachioplasty procedure in which the scar extends into the underarm area, often onto the chest wall.

brachioplasty, short-scar: a brachioplasty procedure in which the scar is limited to the upper one-third of the inner arm and axilla.

brachioplasty, standard: a brachioplasty procedure in which the scar runs along the inner arm, often into the axilla.

breast augmentation: a surgical procedure that increases the size or alters the shape of breasts through the use of prosthetic implants.

breast implant: a saline or silicone-filled prosthetic device.

breast lift: a surgical procedure that reshapes the breast and lifts the nipple to a more youthful position by removal of excess skin.

breast ptosis: sagging of the breasts as defined by the level of the nipple in relation to the inframammary crease.

breast reduction: a surgical procedure that reduces the size of the breasts.

buttock augmentation: a surgical procedure that increases the size of the buttocks.

buttock lift: a surgical procedure that removes excess skin, and possibly fat, from the buttocks.

cannula: a hollow metal instrument used for liposuction.

capsular contracture: abnormal scar tissue formation around a breast implant.

cardiologist: a medical doctor specializing in treatment of the heart.

catabolism: the phase of metabolism in which the complex materials of living tissue are broken down for release of energy.

cellulite: the dimpled or puckered appearance of skin due to the way underlying adipose tissue is suspended.

cervicoplasty: neck lift.

chemical peel: application of a caustic chemical to remove the outer layer of skin and allow for regeneration with a new layer.

cholecystectomy: gallbladder removal.

circulating nurse: an operating room nurse working outside of the sterile operating field.

cohesive gel: type of silicone used in newer generation silicone breast implants.

cold compresses: soft, thick, absorbent cloth, or several layers of cloth, first dipped in cold water and then wrung out, placed directly on a swollen part of the body to reduce swelling and provide temporary relief.

collagen: a strong, fibrous protein found in skin, ligaments, bone, cartilage, and other tissue. Skin elasticity relies on the integrity of collagen present in the skin.

complete blood count (CBC): a blood test to check the number of red blood cells, white blood cells, platelets and hemoglobin level.

complication: an undesirable effect of treatment that can change the outcome and may require additional treatment.

comprehensive metabolic panel (CMP): a group of fourteen blood tests used to evaluate organ function and to check for conditions such as diabetes, kidney and liver disease.

compression garment: a garment that is stretchy or adjustable and that is worn after surgery to aid in the healing process.

connective tissue: the tissue which binds together and is the support of the various structures of the body; components include strands of collagen and elastic fibers.

consultation: the first meeting with a plastic surgeon, when a patient learns about contouring procedures.

contour: the outline of a shape or form.

cosmetic surgery: the surgical reshaping of normal structures of the body.

deep vein thrombosis (DVT): a blood clot that forms in a major vein of the legs, pelvis, or arms.

deflation: refers to volume loss in body areas such as the breasts, arms, thighs, and buttocks (due to the loss of fat and atrophy of glandular tissue or muscle).

dehiscence: separation of wound edges.

depressive disorder: any of several disabling depressive illnesses, including major depression, characterized by prolonged periods of deep sadness, persistent feelings of hopelessness, loss of interest in activities, marked decrease in energy, and possibly other symptoms.

dermabrasion: a skin resurfacing procedure that uses a rotating wire brush, or a similar tool, to sand off the top layer of skin, causing a new layer of skin to grow that is smoother and has fewer blemishes.

dermatitis: a general term for any inflammation of the skin characterized by itching, swelling, or redness.

dermis: the inner layer of skin.

diabetes: a disease in which blood glucose is high.

dog ear: a mound of excess skin located at the end of an incision.

drains *or* drainage tubes: small, plastic tubes that are inserted into surgical incisions towards the end of a procedure to drain any accumulating fluids after surgery.

dressings: bandages that are placed on or wrapped around regions of the body that were contoured to absorb excess fluid and protect incisions.

eczema: a skin disorder characterized by itching and inflammation.

edema: swelling caused by fluid retention in tissues of the body.

elastin: a connective tissue protein responsible for the skin's flexibility and elasticity.

elective surgery: a planned, non-emergency surgical procedure.

electrocautery: a technique applied during surgical procedures to stop bleeding, using a small probe with an electrical current.

electrolytes: minerals such as sodium and potassium that regulate bodily functions.

endotracheal tube (ETT): a plastic tube inserted through the mouth into the windpipe to assist with breathing.

epidermis: the outer layer of skin.

epinephrine: same as adrenaline. Often used in plastic surgery to constrict blood vessels which minimizes blood loss.

excess skin: hanging, sagging, or redundant skin that has lost its elasticity and cannot retract even through rigorous exercising. Getting rid of it involves a surgical body contouring procedure.

extension: the motion of straightening out.

face lift: a surgical procedure that rejuvenates the lower two-thirds of the face.

fascia: a tough fibrous membrane that usually surrounds muscles and various organs.

fascial plication: repair of rectus diastasis by suturing of the fascia to tighten the abdominal muscles.

fat: a kind of body tissue that stores energy.

fatty acids: the basic chemical units of fat.

FDA: the Food and Drug Administration, the governmental agency that regulates food, drugs, supplements, and medical devices in the United States.

fibrin glue: a type of surgical tissue adhesive derived from human products.

flexion: the motion of bending.

forearm: portion of the arm from the elbow to the wrist

forehead lift: a surgical procedure that reduces the appearance of forehead wrinkles and rejuvenates the upper portion of a person's face.

gastric bypass: a type of weight loss surgery that reduces the stomach to a small pouch and allows food to bypass a portion of the digestive system in order to minimize the body's intake of calories.

gastroplasty: a surgical weight loss procedure in which the stomach is made smaller with the use of staples.

general anesthesia: the administration of a drug that leaves a patient unconscious and free of pain during a surgical procedure.

gynecomastia: abnormally large male breasts.

gynecoid body type: pear-shaped figure.

hematoma: a collection or pocket of blood caused by a bleeding vessel which may require surgical drainage.

hemoglobin: the molecule in a red blood cell that carries oxygen.

hemophilia: an inherited bleeding disorder.

hematologist: a blood specialist.

heparin: a drug that thins the blood and prevents clot formation.

hernia: a protrusion of an organ or tissue through an opening in the wall of the cavity in which it is contained.

high blood pressure: persistent elevation of blood pressure above the normal range.

hypertrophic scar: abnormal scar formation in which the scar is widened or raised.

hypertrophy: an increase in the size of an organ or tissue.

infection: an inflammation or illness caused by invading organisms, such as bacteria.

informed consent: A process in which a patient, or a parent or guardian, is informed of the potential risks, benefits and alternatives of a surgery or other treatment and legally agrees to accept those risks.

inframmary fold: the crease below the breast.

inner thigh lift: a contouring procedure that removes excess skin, and possibly excess fat along the inner aspect of the thigh.

intertriginous: a fold where there is skin-to-skin contact.

intravenous (IV): administration of a fluid or drug directly into a vein.

jowl: sagging of the lower face evident at the jawline.

keloid: an abnormal scar which has grown beyond the initial site of a surgical incision or injury.

laparoscopy: performing a procedure within the abdominal cavity using small incisions and the aid of a specialized camera.

laser resurfacing: using light of a certain wavelength to remove the outer layer of skin to allow for regeneration with a new layer.

lateral: towards the side of the body.

laxity: looseness.

lidocaine: a local anesthetic.

lipectomy: the excision of adipose or fatty tissue.

lipectomy, abdominal: another term for abdominoplasty.

lipectomy, circumferential: another term for a body lift.

lipectomy, suction-assisted (SAL): liposuction.

lipoplasty: liposuction.

liposuction: removing fat tissue below the skin using a suctioning process.

local anesthesia: the injection of a drug that blocks pain sensation at the site of a surgical procedure.

love handles: collection of fat above the hip bones which extend around the side of the body.

lower arm: the part of the arm that extends below the elbow.

lymphedema: swelling from accumulation of fluid within tissues, often in the legs.

macromastia: oversize of the female breast.

malabsorption: abnormal absorption of nutrients from the digestive tract.

malnourishment: a state of bad or poor nutrition, in which the body is not receiving enough nutrients to resist infection, repair damage and provide for growth and development.

mammogram: an x-ray method used to evaluate and screen breast tissue for cancer and other abnormalities.

markings: lines, arrows, symbols, and other writings made with a marking pen directly on the skin by a plastic surgeon prior to surgery. These markings help direct the surgeon during the procedure.

massive weight loss: in general, weight reduction in excess of one hundred pounds.

mastopexy: breast lift.

mastopexy, anchor: a breast lift method that uses an anchor-shaped incision for breasts that sag significantly.

mastopexy, concentric: also known as a periareolar mastopexy, circumareolar mastopexy or "doughnut mastopexy", a breast lift technique that uses a circular incision around the areola.

mastopexy, crescent: a breast lift method that uses a semi-circular incision around the areola for breasts that sag only mildly.

mastopexy, vertical: a breast lift technique that uses an incision around the areola and a vertical incision from the areola to the inframammary fold.

medial thighplasty: an inner thigh lift.

medial thighplasty, horizontal: the traditional inner thigh lift in which the scar runs along the groin crease.

medial thighplasty, modified or short scar: an inner thigh lift in which the vertical scar is limited to the upper one-third of the inner thigh. There may also be a horizontal scar.

medial thighplasty, vertical: an inner thigh lift in which a vertical scar extends the entire length of the inner thigh to the level of the knee. There may also be a horizontal scar.

mesh: a synthetic screen-like material used for hernia repair.

metabolism: the process of building the body's complex structures from nutrients (anabolism) and breaking them down for energy production (catabolism).

mineral: a nutrient such as calcium or iron necessary to maintain health.

monsplasty: surgical contouring of the pubic area.

mons pubis: medical term for pubic area.

mons pubis ptosis: sagging of the pubic area.

morbid obesity: having a BMI of forty or above or being at least one hundred pounds above ideal weight.

morbidity: an undesired result or complication.

mortality: refers to death.

myocardial infarction: a heart attack.

narcotic: an opiate medication used for treatment of pain.

nasolabial fold: a skin crease extending from the nose to the corner of the mouth.

neck lift: a surgical procedure that improves the definition and appearance of the

neck by removing excess skin and fat and tightening underlying muscles.

necrosis: pertaining to the death of skin or other tissues.

neoumbilicoplasty: surgical creation of a belly button.

nicotine: a substance found in cigarette smoke and all tobacco products. Harmful to humans and other living organisms, nicotine significantly increases surgical risks and impairs the skin's healing process.

non-absorbable sutures: surgical stitches that do not dissolve on their own.

nutrition: the food and liquid required to maintain life and health.

obese: being above normal weight and having a BMI greater than 30.

open bariatric procedure: a surgical weight loss procedure performed through a standard vertical incision down the midline of the abdomen. The incision is significantly longer than the one centimeter incisions used for a laparoscopic approach.

oral: by mouth.

outpatient: a patient who receives care at a medical facility, not extending beyond twenty four hours.

osteomalacia: softening of the bones due to vitamin D deficiency.

osteoporosis: a decrease in bone density with an increased risk for fracture.

outer thigh lift: a surgical contouring procedure that removes excess skin, and possibly excess fat, tightening the outer thigh area.

overweight: being above normal weight and having a BMI between 25 and 30.

panniculectomy: a surgical procedure that removes the pannus from the abdominal region. Does not involve fascial plication.

pannus: a large "apron" of skin hanging over the abdomen, due to obesity and usually made worse with weight loss. Also called an *abdominal panniculus.*

partial thromboplastin time (PTT): a test that measures blood clotting ability; used to measure the effect of heparin, a blood thinner.

patient-controlled analgesia: a method of pain control in which the patient self-administers a preset dose of pain medication.

pectoral muscle: chest muscle.

plastic surgeon: a medical doctor specializing in reconstructive and cosmetic surgical procedures to improve function and/or appearance of a body part.

platelet: a type of blood cell involved in blood clot formation.

platysma: a broad and thin muscle that covers the neck area.

platysmaplasty: surgical repair of the neck muscle (platysma) to provide better contour with elimination of visible bands in the neck.

plication: in body contouring surgery, the process of tightening muscle or fascia with sutures.

pneumonia: inflammation or infection in the lungs.

post-operative instructions: a set of instructions provided by the plastic surgeon for a patient to follow after surgery to minimize pain and complications, maximize the success of the procedure, and help the recovery period go smoothly.

postoperative garment: a special type of elastic attire worn after surgery which provides support and comfort and aids in the healing process.

prophylactic: preventative.

prosthesis: an artificial device used to represent or replace a body part.

prothrombin time (PT): a test that measures blood clotting ability; used to measure the effect of warfarin.

ptosis: droop or sagging.

pulmonary embolism (PE): a blood clot which has lodged in the lung, usually originating as a deep venous thrombosis.

pulmonologist: a medical doctor specializing in treatment of the lungs.

reconstructive surgery: surgery performed on an abnormal body structure to restore or improve function or to approximate a normal appearance.

recommended dietary allowance (RDA): a calculated average daily intake level for a particular nutrient required for healthy individuals, which varies according to age and gender.

rectus diastasis: separation of abdominal muscles.

rectus abdominus muscles: the abdominal muscles which are separated in rectus diastasis.

red blood cell: the cell that carries oxygen to tissues in the body.

reduction mammaplasty: a breast reduction procedure.

relapse: recurrence of tissue sagging, often earlier than expected.

revisional surgery: repeat or secondary surgery to correct, modify or improve results from a previous procedure.

residency training: years of advanced training for doctors after medical school. This hands-on medical specialty training is done in a hospital or similar setting working alongside senior doctors.

rhytid: skin wrinkle.

rhytidectomy: face lift.

rippling: a wrinkled or rippled appearance at the skin surface due to an underlying breast implant.

saddle bag: fat collection along the outer thigh area.

saline: a salt-water solution.

scar: a permanent mark left from healing of a wound due to surgery or an injury.

scar contracture: scar shortening which can distort surrounding tissue or limit motion.

scar migration: change in position of a scar, often due to recurrent skin looseness and the effects of gravity.

scrub nurse: a member of the sterile operating team who prepares and passes instruments and supplies to the surgeon.

self-esteem: a measure of worth or value a person gives himself or herself.

self-image: an individual's perception of himself or herself.

sequential compression device (SCD): a device worn on the lower extremities to minimize the chance for deep venous thrombosis.

seroma: an accumulation of straw-colored fluid beneath the skin.

serum: the clear liquid part of blood.

silicone: a synthetic material often used in implantable medical devices and derived from silica, a substance found abundantly in nature.

skin elasticity: the property of skin that determines how well it springs back after being pulled, stretched, or pinched.

sleep apnea: a temporary absence of breathing during sleep.

slough: to shed or cast off.

SMAS: short for superficial musculoaponeurotic system, a sheet of connective tissue below the skin of the face.

soft tissue filler: injection of a filler material such as fat or collagen beneath the skin to smooth wrinkles.

staging: in body contouring surgery, the planning of multiple procedures over time.

standing cone: medical term for dog ear, a mound of excess skin located at the end of an incision.

sterile: free from living microorganisms.

steroid: a type of drug used to relieve swelling and inflammation.

striae: skin stretch marks.

subcutaneous layer: the layer found beneath skin which contains fat and connective tissue.

subglandular: refers to placement of a breast implant below the breast tissue and above the chest muscle.

submentoplasty: a neck contouring procedure in which liposuction and platysmaplasty is performed through an incision beneath the chin.

subpectoral: refers to placement of a breast implant below the pectoral muscle.

sun protection factor (SPF): the measure of a sunscreen product's ability to block UV rays. A higher SPF means greater protection.

symmetry: refers to the right and left sides of the body matching perfectly.

thigh lift: a surgical procedure for removing extra skin, and possibly fat, from the outer thighs or inner thighs.

thighplasty: a thigh lift procedure.

torso: the body excluding the head and limbs.

torsoplasty: plastic surgery or contouring of the torso.

torsoplasty, circumferential: another term for a body lift.

trachea: windpipe.

tummy tuck: a surgical contouring procedure that tightens the abdominal wall with fascial plication and removes excess skin and fat.

turkey neck deformity: severe skin sagging of the neck.

twilight sleep: a state reached during anesthesia when there is still a slight degree of consciousness.

umbilicus: belly button.

upper arm: the portion of the arm that extends from the elbow to the shoulder and armpit.

ventral hernia: an abdominal wall hernia.

vital signs: measurements of the body's basic functions, including body temperature, blood pressure, pulse rate, and rate of breathing.

vitamin: a key nutrient necessary for the body to grow and stay healthy.

warfarin: also known as Coumadin; a blood thinner that prevents clot formation.

weight reduction surgery: bariatric surgery.

wetting solution: a saline-based solution important for liposuction which helps minimize blood loss and provides for pain control.

white blood cell: a cell found in blood important for fighting infection and disease.

Z-plasty: a plastic surgery procedure which lengthens a scar to prevent scar contraction which can limit motion.

Index

About the Authors

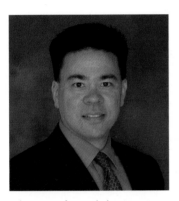

"The journey for weight loss patients can be difficult and challenging at times, but it is one that is life-altering and filled with tremendous health benefits, joy, and satisfaction."

– Dr. Jeffrey L. Sebastian

Jeffrey L. Sebastian, M.D., is a general and plastic surgeon who works extensively with bariatric and massive weight loss patients. In addition to having a private practice in Santa Monica, California, Dr. Sebastian is an assistant clinical professor of surgery at the David Geffen School of Medicine at UCLA and teaches surgery in the Veteran Administration's Greater Los Angeles Healthcare System.

After receiving his bachelor of science degree from the University of California, Los Angeles, Dr. Sebastian attended medical school at the University of California, Davis, where he was elected to the Alpha Omega Alpha Honor Medical Society. He completed training in general surgery and plastic and reconstructive surgery at the UCLA Medical Center, and also completed a fellowship in minimally invasive surgery. Dr. Sebastian is board-certified by the American Board of Surgery (ABS).

He has conducted clinical research in the field of bariatric surgery and pursues research related to stem cells and tissue engineering. Dr. Sebastian has co-authored numerous articles for peer-reviewed medical journals and speaks at state and national conferences pertaining to body contouring after massive weight loss.

Dr. Sebastian may be reached through his Web site: **www.sebastianmd.com.**

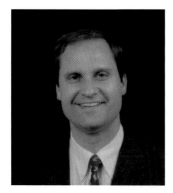

"Body contouring procedures following massive weight loss are usually extremely gratifying for both the patient and surgeon. The results are usually dramatic and provide a significant functional and aesthetic benefit to the patient."

— Dr. Joseph F. Capella

Joseph F. Capella, M.D., is a plastic and reconstructive surgeon in private practice in Ramsey, New Jersey and New York City. He has performed over 3,000 body contouring procedures on patients who have undergone major weight loss. Dr. Capella has been conducting clinical research in surgery for morbid obesity since 1987. He serves on the Post-Bariatric Task Force with the American Society of Plastic Surgeons (ASPS) and has co-authored two books on body contouring after major weight loss.

After receiving his Bachelor of Arts degree from Cornell University in Ithaca, New York, and completing post-graduate studies at Columbia University in New York City, Dr. Capella attended medical school at the State University of New York Health Science Center at Brooklyn. He then completed a residency in general surgery at St. Luke's-Roosevelt Hospital in New York City and a fellowship in plastic and reconstructive surgery at the Mayo Clinic in Minnesota.

Dr. Capella is certified by the American Board of Surgery (ABS) and the American Board of Plastic Surgery (ABPS). He is a fellow of the American College of Surgeons and a clinical assistant professor of surgery at the University of Medicine and Dentistry of New Jersey at Newark.

He frequently lectures on body contouring techniques at national and international plastic surgery conferences. He has appeared as an expert guest on several television shows including 20/20 and The View. Dr. Capella has co-authored numerous articles for medical journals and teaches courses about post-bariatric body contouring to fellow surgeons.

Dr. Capella may be reached through his Web site: **www.capellaplasticsurgery.net**.

J. **Peter Rubin, M.D.**, is a general and plastic surgeon at the University of Pittsburgh Medical Center (UPMC) in Pittsburgh, Pennsylvania. He is founder and director of UPMC's Life After Weight Loss, an innovative program dedicated to meeting plastic surgery needs of the bariatric patient after weight loss, with special emphasis placed on nutritional and lifestyle counseling. Dr. Rubin also is director of the Adipocyte Biology Laboratory and co-director of the Aesthetic Plastic Surgery Center at UPMC.

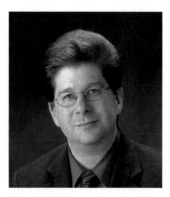

"For many, body contouring completes the weight loss journey. My goal is to integrate key lifestyle components with innovative surgical procedures in order to help patients reach their goals."

—Dr. J. Peter Rubin

He received his undergraduate degree from Grinnell College in Iowa and attended medical school at Tufts University in Boston, Massachusetts. Dr. Rubin completed residency training in plastic surgery at Harvard University in Boston. He has done research on the safety of anesthetic techniques for liposuction, tissue engineering of adipose tissue, xenotransplantation, and other areas.

Board-certified with the American Board of Surgery (ABS) and the American Board of Plastic Surgery (ABPS), Dr. Rubin specializes in body contouring following massive weight loss and breast reconstruction. He serves on the American Society of Plastic Surgery's (ASPS) Bariatric Task Force, which develops safety guidelines and educational programs. Recently he was appointed as the first official liaison between the ASPS and the American Society of Bariatric Surgery.

Dr. Rubin is assistant professor of surgery at the University of Pittsburgh School of Medicine. He frequently lectures at national meetings about liposuction safety and his work with gastric bypass patients. He is published in a number of peer-reviewed medical journals.

Dr. Rubin may be reached through this Web site: **lifeafterweightloss.upmc.com**.

Consumer Health Titles from Addicus Books

Visit our online catalog at www.AddicusBooks.com

Organizations, associations, corporations, hospitals, and other groups may qualify for special discounts when ordering more than 24 copies. For more information, please contact the Special Sales Department at Addicus Books. Phone (402) 330-7493.
Email: info@AddicusBooks.com

Please send:

_____copies of_____
(Title of book)

at $_____each   TOTAL: _____

Nebraska residents add 5% sales tax   _____

Shipping/Handling
$4.00 postage for first book.
$1.10 postage for each additional book   _____

   TOTAL ENCLOSED: _____

Name _____

Address _____

City_____State_____Zip _____

☐ **Visa**   ☐ **MasterCard**   ☐ **American Express**

Credit card number _____Expiration date _____

Order by credit card, personal check or money order. Send to:

Addicus Books
Mail Order Dept.
P.O. Box 45327
Omaha, NE 68145
Or, order **TOLL FREE: 800-352-2873**
or online at
www.AddicusBooks.com